COUNTY

COUNTY

LIFE, DEATH AND POLITICS AT CHICAGO'S PUBLIC HOSPITAL

DAVID A. ANSELL, MD, MPH

ACADEMY CHICAGO PUBLISHERS

Published by Academy Chicago Publishers
An imprint of Chicago Review Press, Incorporated
814 North Franklin Street
Chicago, Illinois 60610

ISBN 978-089733-719-9

Library of Congress Cataloging-in-Publication Data
Ansell, David, MD.
County : life, death, and politics at Chicago's public hospital / by David Ansell.
        p. ; cm.
ISBN 978-0-89733-719-9 (paperback)
1. Cook County Hospital (Chicago, Ill.)—History. 2. County hospitals—
Illinois—Chicago—History. 3. Physicians—Chicago—Autobiography.
I. Title. [DNLM: 1. Cook County Hospital. (Chicago, Ill.)
2. Physicians—Chicago—Autobiography. 3. History, 20th Century—Chicago.
4. Hospitals, County—history—Chicago. 5. Internship and Residency—Chicago—
Autobiography. WZ 100]
RA982.C452A57 2010
362.1109773'1—dc22
2010053279

Cover design: Joan Sommers Design
Front cover images: (Top) Wheelchairs in the Emergency Room, Cook County Hospital
(Courtesy Gordy Schiff, MD); (Bottom) Operating Room, Cook County Hospital (Courtesy
Cook County Health and Hospital System Archives)
Pages 8–9: Cook County Hospital, 1914 (Courtesy Cook County Health and Hospital System
Archives)

www.countythebook.com

Printed in the United States of America

CONTENTS

This book is dedicated to those individuals who, because of their race, income, immigrant status or lack of health insurance, have been denied the most basic of health services that should have been available to them as a simple condition of their humanity.

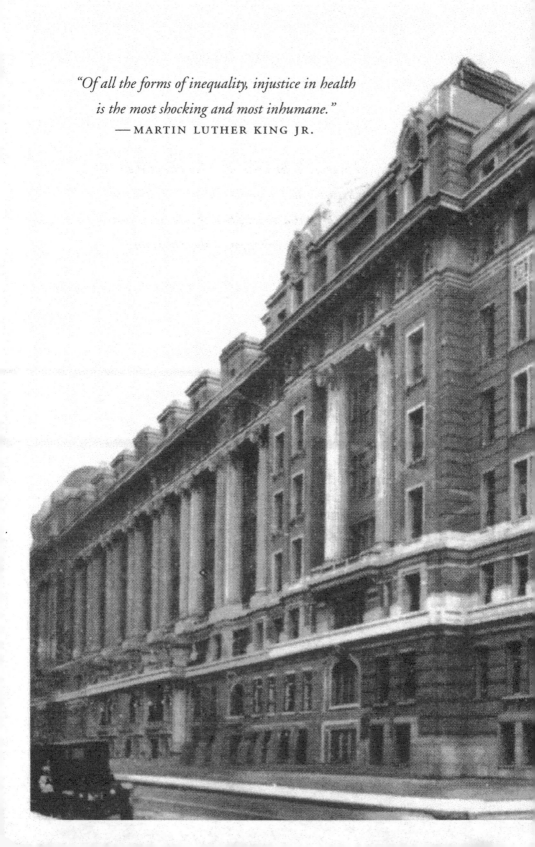

"*Of all the forms of inequality, injustice in health is the most shocking and most inhumane.*"
— MARTIN LUTHER KING JR.

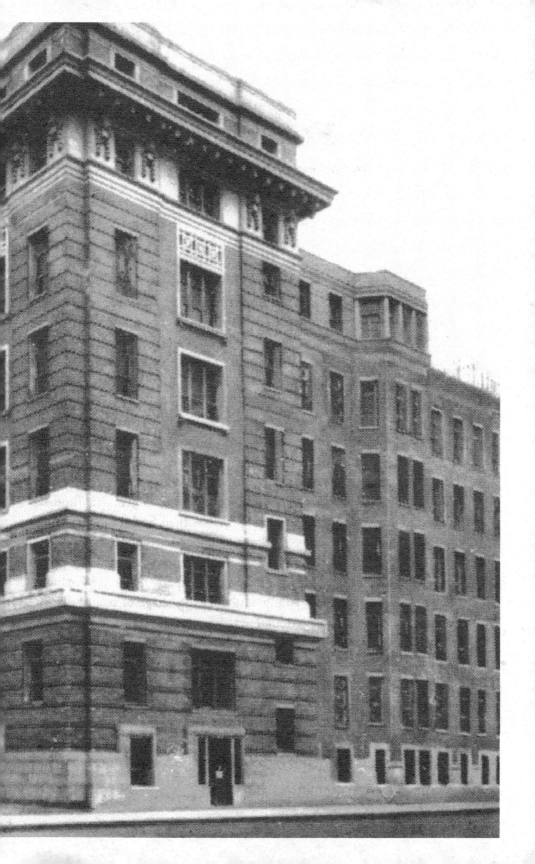

Foreword

TO THE FIRST PAPERBACK EDITION

IN THE TWO YEARS since the publication of *County: Life, Death and Politics at Chicago's Public Hospital*, the health care landscape in the U.S. has changed dramatically. In March 2010, the Patient Protection and Affordable Care Act was passed in Congress and signed into law by President Barack Obama. Two years later, in June 2012, after a series of lower court skirmishes, the Supreme Court of the United States upheld the central tenets of the legislation and the largest piece of social legislation in the US, since the passage of Medicare and Medicaid in 1965, became the undisputed law of the land.

About half of the newly insured will be adults living below the poverty line, who will receive their coverage through their state funded Medicaid plans. The other half will purchase their health insurance on newly established insurance marketplaces, where insurance companies will compete for enrollees. U.S. citizens are now mandated to purchase health insurance or face a fine. Other aspects of the law include new provisions that allow young adults up to the age of twenty-six to remain covered on their parents' health insurance policies. Children and adults with pre-existing health conditions can no longer be denied coverage. All insured Americans can access preventive health care without co-payments as a component of what has been called "essential health benefits." Finally, insurance companies are limited to claiming no more than twenty percent of their costs for administrative overhead or profit. It all sounds like good news for those who have toiled for meaningful health-care reform for years. But, for many of us who have battled for a single-payer health care system in the United States, one that treats all Americans equally, regardless of ability to pay, the cup is half full.

As a starter, the Affordable Care Act will leave as many as twenty-five million people without health insurance, about as many as there were in the early 1980s. The most significant flaw in the Affordable Care Act is that it perpetuates the tiered health care system in the US that depends on expensive private insurance companies and fragmented state Medicaid systems to deliver separate and unequal health care in parallel systems, for rich and poor. Thirty-five years ago, these separate and unequal conditions beckoned my friends and me to join other young doctors and nurses at Chicago's Cook County Hospital, the legendary public hospital on Chicago's West Side. It was the perpetuation of health care inequality in Chicago and across the U.S. that prompted me, many years later, to write this book.

I have had the perfect perspective to write about health care inequality. In my three decades as a doctor in Chicago, I have worked at three Chicago health care institutions along one Chicago road: Ogden Avenue. Once an ancient Native-American trail, it cuts a swath across Chicago's West Side and these three hospitals sit within one mile of each other. From my perspective as a Chicago physician and health care disparity researcher turned hospital administrator and from the experiences of my patients who followed me up and down Ogden Avenue as I moved from hospital to hospital, you could not invent a more unequal health care system in America than my patients and I have found along this one street in Chicago.

I have described my experiences as a doctor in Chicago and that of my patients as "three hospitals, one street and two worlds." It was not the doctors, not the nurses nor the administrators who made these three institutions and access to quality care so variable, but rather the financing of the US health care system itself. I had an encounter with the Chief Medical Officer of Cook County Hospital not long after *County* was published. "David," he said to me in the fall of 2011, as we sat at a table in a dining room at Rush University Medical Center, the private academic medical center across the street from the County Hospital, "The waiting list for the eye clinic at County Hospital is so long that a patient can go blind waiting to be examined." At Rush, just a few hundred yards away from the public hospital's eye clinic, a patient with the right insurance card could see an ophthalmologist the same day. These health care inequalities are not just the subject for arcane public policy debates. They are literally a matter of life and death. Much has been written about the growing wealth inequalities in the United States, but the idea that someone could die earlier because of poverty or lack of a proper insurance card, violates the core American principles of fairness, equal rights and choice. Unfortunately, the Affordable Care Act will perpetuate these health care inequalities.

Chicago is the ever-present protagonist in this story: infamous for its historic racial segregation, it has been dubbed by the American sociologist, Robert Samson, as the "Great American City" because the conditions within its regional confines speak volumes about the very unresolved inequalities that have splintered American political discourse over the past two centuries. *County* was not intended to be read solely as a memoir, or simply a story about one public hospital in one Midwestern city, but rather as a manifesto about health care inequality in America as viewed though the eyes and experiences of one doctor and his patients from the vantage point of this great American city. On the eve of historic yet flawed health care reform in the U.S., the lessons we learned at Cook County Hospital make me optimistic that we will eventually achieve the kind of single-payer universal health care insurance that our people deserve. As young doctors at Chicago's public hospital we learned never to take no as an answer when a patient's life was on the line. And so it is now with the nation's health care at stake. Winston Churchill said about Americans, "Americans always do the right thing, after exhausting all other possibilities." It is time for us to do the right thing.

— David A. Ansell, MD, MPH
   Chicago, Illinois
   April 2013

Introduction

COOK COUNTY HOSPITAL, Chicagoland's monstrous public hospital, has at least three functions. Its first, and arguably most important role, is political, for party-favored contractors and employees and, not least, as a last resort for poor patients. "County" (as it came to be known) played a crucial role in the health care delivery system by being the caregiver to the poor, a demographic that is—and increasingly so—African American, Mexican, Puerto Rican, and immigrant. Finally, County has had a huge role in the training of physicians and other health professionals in the entire region. For more than a century and a half, County has had an immense presence in both the medical scene and the larger political and sociological life of its community. Over the years, no author has succeeded in writing the story of this colossal venture. Several explanations of this failure come to mind, from simple lack of literary skill, to a propensity to write anecdotal, personal diaries. Past authors failed to link County's fortunes to the world-historic medical and social events that emerged in this time frame. To name but a few: the discovery and application of anesthetics; the proof of germ etiologies, followed by description of viruses; antibiotics; immunization; vaccination; and ever more invasive surgeries to heart, lungs and brain. County, with its vast patient population, was a perfect setting for clinical trials that facilitated many of these advances. Writing the definitive story looked like an impossible task. At least half a dozen authors over the years sought to capture the reality of Cook County Hospital. Overall, many authors displayed an inability to relate its century-and-a-half history to the spectacular transformation of bioscience and medical care in this same period. David Ansell has done it. He has captured the County story vividly and comprehensively. His own career is just the right preparation for this task: four years of training to be an internist in the County's Department of Medicine, another thirteen years as an attending physician at Cook County Hospital, then ten years of service in the city's major private hospital caring for the poor, Mount Sinai Hospital, and, lately, Medical Director at the prestigious Rush University Medical Center. All this, capped by his selection to serve on the newly-created independent governing board in charge of the Cook County Health and Hospital System. Given the dire straits of our public hospitals— underfunding, closures, uninsured patients—this fine book could be a dirge, or a celebration. In any event, it is an authentic and accurate description of a most consequential chapter in our country's history, and a reflection on our nation's failure, unlike the other major western industrialized nations, to make equal access to health care a right for all.

— Quentin Young, MD
Chicago, January 2011

PROLOGUE

The Hospital

IN THE SPRING OF 1978, five newly-minted medical school graduates loaded all of our belongings into a twenty-four foot U-Haul Truck and trekked from Syracuse, New York to Chicago, Illinois to begin internships at Cook County Hospital. A little more than two years prior to our arrival, the hospital was the site of the longest doctor strike in U.S. history when the House Staff Union we were about to join walked out over the intolerable patient care conditions at the hospital. The strike ended when the hospital agreed to some of the patient care improvements that the young doctors demanded. However, seven of the House Staff leaders, doctors no older than we were, were sentenced to Cook County Jail for defying a back-to-work order. The Cook County Hospital we were about to enter was a simmering cauldron of conflict and third-world patient care. We came to County Hospital eyes wide open because of its troubles, not in spite of them. We did not come to County Hospital just to learn to be doctors. We came to County because we believed that health care was a right, not a privilege. That as doctors we had to lead the fight for fairness, equity and universal health care in the U.S. Cook County Hospital was at the front lines of this battle. We encountered roadblocks: an antiquated facility; inept management; underfunding; a corrupt political Machine; patients who were dumped and refused care at other hospitals; our own inadequacies as doctors; patients who died at our doorstep or on our watches.

In the 160 years since its doors first opened, Cook County Hospital has been an institution of epic medical achievements. It was the birthplace of America's first blood bank. Home of America's first trauma unit. Its wards had been graced by some of the greatest doctors in the history of American medicine. For a century, until the 1960s, County boasted one of the most competitive internships in the country. It inspired physicians to pay and compete for the privilege of attending there. It was also a troubled institution from its inception and struggled with the same underfunding, poor management and political interference we encountered more than a century later.

By the 1960s a unique set of circumstances placed Cook County Hospital at the center of the national debate about race and health in the U.S. It was simply that Cook County Hospital was in the right place at the right time. As Chicago's black population quadrupled from 250,000 to over one million in the years between 1930 and 1960, racial segregation of neighborhoods and institutions limited black choices for everything from jobs to schools to hospitals. County Hospital became the de-facto hospital for black people in Chicago. By 1960, County was serving the black community and an immigrant Mexican community almost exclusively. In fact, in this decade, eighty percent of Chicago's black births and fifty percent of all black deaths were at County Hospital. This was not just an issue of poverty. Many of the black patrons at County had well-paying jobs and health insurance.

Racial segregation was actively enforced and many Chicago hospitals refused to serve black patients until laws like the Hill-Burton Act and Medicare-mandated desegregation. The presence of the County Hospital allowed for the extraordinary exclusion of black patients from almost all the other hospitals. This was a form of Jim Crow as heinous as any practiced in the Deep South and enforced, not by law, but by the collective behavior of an entire city's establishment. Ultimately, this legacy of segregated care in the under-resourced public system contributed fifty years later to the gaping black-white racial disparities in health outcomes for which Chicago is notorious. Professor Pierre de Vise, a Chicago reform Democrat, criticized County Hospital in the late 1960s as "this criminal concentration of medical care for the million people who are shut out of the private health system" and as "a major factor in the death each year of approximately 1,000 Chicagoans."

By the late 1960s the conditions at the hospital had deteriorated badly under the strain of the growing black population and its health needs. Beds lined up two to three in the hallways. Over 1,000 emergency visits and fifty births each day. This was in the same United States that had just landed a man on the moon. The demands for improvements and change reached full throttle but fell on the deaf ears of a recalcitrant white political establishment. It was a time of social change in Chicago and the country and a new breed of activist doctors and nurses began to organize for improvements within the soot-covered walls of County. The long-time superintendent of the hospital who had been a fixture there since 1914 retired in 1967. A militant black community along with these activist doctors and nurses, many of whom had come of age during the civil rights movement in the U.S., demanded a change of governance to a professional and independent board. In response, the state legislature wrested control of Cook County Hospital away from the Democratic Machine which ran all Cook County government and handed it to a newly constituted independent Governing Commission in the hopes of improving care. But governance change was not enough. The funding of hospital services was insufficient to improve conditions. The Democratic Machine blocked the Governing Commission from gaining fiscal control over the hospital and by the late 1970s the Governing Commission was unable to manage supply shortages and labor unrest at the hospital. The conflict between the County Board and the Governing Commission would explode within a year of our arrival.

The County Hospital we arrived at in 1978 was ground zero for all the crucial questions facing the U.S. health care system. What is the best way to fund and deliver health care to the poor and uninsured?

Can separate health care delivery systems, one for the insured and one for the uninsured, ever be fair or equal? What is our nation's commitment to closing the racial gap in American life spans? How do institutions such as Cook County Hospital contribute to these racial gaps? Little did I know, thirty years later, I would be sitting on the Board of Directors of this very institution asking these same crucial questions. The story of this singular public hospital is the story of health care in America, and its travails speak to our national failure to declare that heath care is a right and that Americans should not face early death or disability because they are uninsured. This is my story but could be the story of any number of young doctors and nurses who came to Cook County Hospital to join in a battle for health equity that thirty years later has yet to be won.

— David Ansell, MD, MPH
   Chicago, January 2011

CHAPTER 1

1989: You Should Write That Book

"You'd never want to wake up and find yourself in Cook County Hospital, the nation's first and oldest public hospital. The building looks as huge, grey and battered as a vanquished and abandoned old battleship run aground on the shattered streets just west of Chicago's Loop. The hallways and waiting rooms—there's no nicer way to put this—are thick with sick people who have also run aground and seem abandoned to waiting, limping, straining, coughing, sighing and sweating, bleeding, crying."

—Scott Simon, *Weekend Edition*, National Public Radio, 1994

I BOLTED DOWN THE STEPS from the General Medicine Clinic at Cook County Hospital. My scuffed, brown Rockports smacked the concrete stairs as my right palm skimmed the handrail, its blue paint, once bright and cheery now worn to its steely base by thousands of hands, perhaps as tardy as mine. I was late. I was always late. A major weakness and character flaw—one I am still trying to mend years later. Late, because I stuffed my life, like the overflowing shopping carts of the scavengers who loitered on Madison Street. A victim of both my idealism and impatience. The cacophony and chaos of County Hospital made a perfect setting for my appetite. It was an "all you can eat" kind of place. It was barely 1:00 p.m. and I was gorged.

I spent the morning seeing patients in the clinic; the door was full of charts; the waiting room stuffed as tight as a stockyard cattle car. The last patient had taken me longer than I hoped and after I packed her off with her prescriptions and laboratory orders, I wrote a hasty note in the chart, looked at my watch and cursed. I grabbed my stethoscope from the desk, shoved it into the front pocket of my corduroys and raced to the stairwell.

I punched open the door at the bottom of the stairs and was whisked into a vortex of patients traversing the hallway, a whirring of sounds and the vaguely pungent and familiar odor of musk and oiled hair. If I was going to make it to my meeting, I needed to do my best Walter Payton impression and slice through this gauntlet without being thwarted by the doctors, staff and passersby who bustled past the waiting room of the sprawling Ambulatory Screening Clinic. Every day, 200 to 300 unscheduled patients swarmed through its doors seeking medical attention. Today, like every other day, it was more mosh pit than clinic. The cumulative body heat of the masses overwhelmed the air conditioning system's attempt to cool the room.

As I began my cut through the winding corridor, my final dash to the meeting, a voice intercepted me, the clipped Arabic-tinged English of a colleague, Iraqi-born kidney specialist, Dr. Asad Bakir, an island of calm amid the erupting first floor of Fantus Clinic. I turned. His hair was combed in a neat part, each strand obedient and in place on his head in contrast to my roiling mop of curls. His starched gray laboratory coat and Armani-style trousers were pristine, their creases sharp as a razor's edge. I sighed. My shoulders slumped. I'd never make the meeting. I stopped and shook his hand. I liked Bakir. Eight years earlier I had worked with him when I was a resident in training and he wrote on my evaluation that I should be considered for a spot as an attending physician at County, perhaps the highest endorsement a resident could receive. We were both distracted by a crushing assemblage of patients and doctors and we gawked like sightseers.

"You know, David," he said in the British public school accent and rolled r's so typical of Iraqis of his age, as his eyes darted across the crowd in the waiting area in awe, "Someone should wrrr-ite a book about this place." The conditions at Cook County Hospital were so appalling and the suffering of such magnitude that we often felt that

if the outside world knew about it, there would be more outcry to end
or improve it.

"Actually," I replied, "I plan to write a book, I'm just not sure anyone would believe it." My assertion was interrupted by a registration
clerk's frantic call.

"Dr. Ansell! There's a man down in the men's washroom!" I hes-
itated before I pounced into action. And not only because I would
now surely miss my meeting. The men's washroom was about thirty
feet away. Its reputation for filth was legendary at County, with just
two stalls to accommodate the thousands of patients and staff who
waited or passed by every day. Add to that a spotty cleaning schedule,
the semi-sweet odor of ancient urine deposits left by a multitude of
bladder-challenged Chicagoans and the tags of competing West Side
gangs carved on every available surface, and you had one place I never
deigned to enter in all my years at County.

Bakir and I exchanged a "let's roll" glance. I tore past the vend-
ing-machine-lined back wall of Fantus accompanied by the drum roll
clickety-clack back beat of Bakir's loafers on the linoleum. I pushed
through the swinging door of the bathroom and was jolted by an aro-
matic blend of urine, feces and sweat. My heart thumped. On the
floor, visible under the closed door of the first stall was the limp body
of a man in the fetal position. I seized the stall door and shook it.
Locked from within. No time to waste. I slammed open the adjacent
stall and scaled the toilet seat, careful not to plunge my feet into the
murky water of the bowl below. I grabbed onto the top edge of the
divider between the two stalls with both hands, stretched myself up
on my tippy toes and peeked over. My stethoscope dangled out of my
pants pocket.

"There's a guy down on the floor. He's out cold. Maybe a seizure.
I'm gonna climb over and try to get to him," I said to Bakir below.
With my right foot, stretched as far as it could go on the edge of the
toilet seat, I dragged myself up over the partition, my left foot and leg
flailed and banged on the metal divider between stalls as I grunted
to maneuver over the top. At thirty-seven, I pondered I just might

be a little old for this. Too late. I was committed. Just then, I saw the man twitch. A sign of life. Good news. My foot caught the top of the divider. As I leaned to thrust myself into the other stall, the life-less lump on the floor roared alive, like an outtake from *The Exorcist.* He whipped around toward me, face contorted in fury. A lit cigarette stub with a quarter inch of gray ash dangled between his fingertips. A curlicue of smoke ascended in a lazy waltz up toward me. The man aimed a nicotine stained brown finger at me, as he pried himself up to rest on one elbow.

"Get the fuck out of here!" the homeless man barked, defending his territory. Hanging atop the stall, I struggled to catch my breath. My eyes darted back to Bakir, as I mumbled, "Call security."

I hopped off the toilet and skipped out of the bathroom, brushed my hands together several times, placed them on my thighs and tried to press the crinkles out of my corduroys. Bakir eyed me and shrugged his shoulders as we parted ways.

"You know, David, you should wrr-rite that book."

Twenty-two years have passed since that moment in the bath-room. The same homeless still called County Hospital home. Health reform passed in 2010 to much fanfare. But to many of us grizzled and skeptical veterans of the health-care battles fought on Chicago's West Side, first to save and then transform Cook County Hospital, health reform looked like more of the same. It perpetuates the inequities in our health care system; the very issues we came to County Hospital to challenge. Some things have improved at County Hospital in the thirty-plus years since I came to Chicago, wide-eyed, wild-haired and newly graduated from medical school. On the other hand, many of the problems that I encountered when I arrived there have persisted. And yet County remains a necessary component of the health care safety net because the U.S., unlike most other industrialized nations, does not value equal access to health as a human right.

I owe a big debt to County Hospital. It is where I learned to be a doctor. To diagnose and treat conditions that I had only known as words in a medical school textbook. Taught by other young doctors, as young as I, but also taught by my patients, some of whom still see me so many years later. Most of all, County Hospital is where I first witnessed how unfairness wreaked havoc on my patients' bodies and on their families. How the triad of racism, poverty and lack of insurance conspired to kill my patients and their family members before their time. It is a form of injustice that continues to this day.

CHAPTER 2

1964–1978: Wounded Pigeon Syndrome

"YOU KNOW WHAT'S WRONG WITH YOU?" my dad said, in his east London accent. Here it comes, I thought. My dad had a certain way of berating me and my brothers, able to reduce us to nothing with a word or a glance. However, even his most unkind criticisms reflected a bit of truth. We sat on opposite sides of the kitchen table. The morning light spilled through the windows. It was 1973. I was twenty and home from college. At issue were the bricks I put in all the toilets in my family's house, as a way to reduce water consumption. I didn't tell him. He discovered it weeks later, when he investigated why it was taking multiple flushes to clear his business. He was not happy.

"You've got the wounded pigeon syndrome," he said. Earlier in the year, I had nursed a sick pigeon back to health, an episode that helped my father crystallize what he thought was wrong with me. Wounded pigeon syndrome. He meant that I had a soft spot for the underdog, for farm workers, for the civil rights marchers, for the Vietnamese and for the environment. He did not understand. A generation gap. When I argued with him about some current injustice, he dismissed me with the phrase, "T'was ever thus." This made my blood boil.

I loved my dad, but we did not see eye to eye. He came from a poor East End family in London, the English equivalent to the Lower East Side of New York. And he immigrated with my mom to Binghamton, New York, a white-ethnic shoe factory town on the banks of the mud-colored Susquehanna River in an Appalachian mountain valley, 170 miles from New York City. Binghamton was a sad sack of a city in the midst of a slow death spiral of economic decline. But he found work there, as a doctor in a converted gas station in the country and so he settled. A child of the Depression, he had no time for activism or politics.

He was correct, though. I did have "the wounded pigeon syndrome." My mother's extended Polish family perished in the Holocaust a few years before my birth, and this fact hung over my childhood like the gray fog lingered over a Binghamton morning. I grew up haunted and perhaps even obsessed by the images of the Holocaust. I trace my interest in issues of social justice to my reaction to that horrific event. I was a sensitive kid—"overly sensitive," my mother said. And "weak-chested and knobby-kneed," she'd add if she had your attention. When my family took weekend trips to New York City and we consorted among the throngs along Broadway at night, my brothers and sister ogled the lights. I gaped at the beggars with their cans and signs, some legless on rolling platforms; others who hid in the shadows of alleys, or on the stoops of shuttered businesses, wrapped in layers of clothes. I wanted to help them, to empty my pockets of change and throw it into their tins.

The *CBS Nightly News* thrust 1960s America into our family den. The Kennedy assassinations, and the civil rights and anti-war movements exploded across the black-and-white screen. I was transfixed. Twelve years old during Freedom Summer in 1964, I read the paper in shock as the news of the murders of the three civil rights activists in Mississippi unfolded. The images of Bloody Sunday and the gassing and head-smashing of the civil rights marchers on the Edmund Pettus Bridge in Selma distressed me. By the time student activism burst out in Binghamton in the late 1960s, I was in the thick of it.

Julian Bond, a rising black civil rights leader and the first black person to be elected to the Georgia State Senate since Reconstruction, arrived in town when I was seventeen to lead an anti-war demonstration. I stood on the manicured lawn in front of the copper green-domed Courthouse on a spring day, with my high school posse, wearing an olive green military jacket I had purchased at the local Salvation Army for a few bucks. Bond held forth on racism and the war. Riveted, I listened to him speak as a warm feeling of pride rose from my stomach into my chest, and I realized that I was part of a larger movement that shared my beliefs. I finally had a way to express my feelings about the events in the larger world. We marched against the Vietnam War, winding our way through the working-class Binghamton neighborhoods to jeers and waving American flags. We chanted anti-war slogans in response.

I was asked to write a column in the Binghamton Central High School newspaper during my senior year. "Pa Central," as the column was titled, was supposed to be about school spirit, but in 1969 that was the last thing on my mind. "Expecting William Buckley?" was the sarcastic, anti-authoritarian introduction to my first column. It was not long before I was summoned to the principal's office to explain myself. I stood in front of his desk, hands by my side. He sat looking up at me through horn-rimmed glasses, my newspaper column in front of him, a frown on his face.

"Ansell, what does this mean?" His jowls shook like cow udders, as his index finger tapped in a staccato beat on the paper to make his point. His scalp, visible under his short cropped hair, reddened from front to back like an ink spill on paper. He was a major in the army reserves. Big-boned and closed-minded, he had earlier in the year refused to allow the school to purchase *The Catcher in the Rye* and *Brave New World* for a fiction elective I had arranged with some other seniors. In defiance, we bought our own copies. But he had no problem with our twelfth-grade English required reading of "A letter to my granddaughter about communism," a piece of propaganda by J. Edgar Hoover, the Director of the FBI.

Binghamton Central High School in the late 1960s still bore the remnants of the anti-communist frenzy of the Joseph McCarthy years. Binghamton was a backwater, a town of festering racism and anti-Semitism that seemed impervious to the world outside its mountainous boundaries. Woodstock had been held on a farm about fifty miles away the year before, but it might as well have been in another country.

William Buckley was the national spokesperson of the conservative right, the Glenn Beck of the time, and apparently one of the principal's heroes. My question, "Expecting William Buckley?" irritated him. "This won't do in the school newspaper," he said, and demanded I remove the line. I refused, jaw thrust forward. We argued. I don't know why he relented. I guess I convinced him that the words themselves were innocuous and the double entendre was not so sinister. In the months and weeks that followed, every column I wrote faced the same scrutiny.

The winds of change blasted across the country. Rules and norms were changing quickly. Even at Binghamton Central. The student council had a very strict dress code at my high school. No tee shirts. No sandals. No jeans. No shorts. No culottes. No miniskirts. So I helped organize a vote against the dress code at the student council. "I move we abolish the dress code," I said to the assembled students sitting at school desks in a classroom. "Second," another student chimed in as we had planned. "Any discussion?" The student council advisor blustered and wrung his hands. "You can't do this!" he said. "All in favor? Aye!" the students affirmed. "Against?" Silence. The room broke out in whoops. Gone was the dress code. The next day, Binghamton Central's hallways were a sea of students in tee shirts and jeans, miniskirts and culottes.

By the time I left Binghamton for college in 1970, I was ready to take on the world. College started with the anti-war movement at its peak and ended with the Watergate hearings and Nixon's impeachment. I joined the thousands of college students who marched on Washington in anti-war demonstrations. My friends and I watched the Watergate hearings every day on a flickering, beat-up, black-and-white Zenith, hanging on every revelation. Politics was our lifeblood. The threatened impeachment of Nixon felt like vindication. Like many of my generation, I saw—and still see—activism as a way to improve a flawed world. I chose medicine as a way to channel my altruistic desires to help others. I clung to the hope, naïve perhaps, that health and medicine were free from the conflicts that fractured our larger society.

I was wrong. Four years later, I completed medical school in Syracuse, New York. It was the late 1970s. The activism of the past decade had devolved into a period of stagnation and disillusionment. Medical school felt like a trade school. Maybe it was the juxtaposition of the freewheeling days and social unrest of the sixties and early seventies and the narrow view of disease that characterized the standard medical school curriculum. Women, and, to a lesser degree minorities, were just beginning to be admitted to the medical profession. Chauvinism and anachronistic notions about race and social determinants of disease permeated the classrooms.

I met a group of similarly disgruntled medical students and my wife Paula and I moved with them into an airy old Victorian. Together, through reading and discussions, we developed a perspective on health and society that was absent from our curriculum, one that valued the social etiologies of disease. Some of us developed stress-related symptoms during this period. I had panic attacks that jolted me awake in the night with chest tightness and palpitations that once landed me in an emergency room. For a while I contemplated quitting medical school. Another friend developed strange nerve-related rashes and frightening choking sensations. A third got a duodenal ulcer. We were a flock of wounded pigeons. We decided that we wanted to find a place to train where we could make a difference, where we could confront head-on the social inequities that we believed contributed to ill health, where we could learn medicine in an environment with others like us. There were not many places like this in the U.S. Maybe only one—Cook County Hospital.

CHAPTER 3

1977: Cook County Hospital: We'd Fit Right In

THE COLD CALL TO CHICAGO and the conversation with Mardge Cohen, an intern at Cook County Hospital, clinched it.

"How do you like your internship?" we asked.

"I don't like it!" she said, "I love it!"

We did not know Mardge but discovered her through a mutual contact. Mardge was one of a group of activist medical students, like us, who went to Cook County Hospital to train. Short, with thin brown hair, piercing brown eyes and a Queens accent, she was unabashed in her enthusiasm. Love internship? That was an unexpected response; most residents hated their internship year. Love internship? Mardge's high-decibel endorsement was enough for us. We were determined to visit County Hospital and made an appointment to meet the legendary Chairman of Medicine, Quentin Young.

We drove to Chicago from Syracuse, New York, in my blue Dodge Omni in late 1977, past the vast steel mills that lined the Lake Michigan waterfront from Gary, Indiana, to East Chicago. Billows of white smoke spewed from steel mill smokestacks and the stink of sulfur—the smell of rotten eggs—assaulted our senses. The midnight sky was streaked bubble-gum pink, psychedelic and eerie at the same time. We came to learn, over time, that many of our County patients had migrated from the Jim Crow south to Chicago thirty years earlier to work in those steel mills. Chicago in the late 1970s was not the destination city that it later became. Its reputation had been damaged in the prior decade by white flight, racial and civil unrest. When we arrived it was in a state of decline, as Nelson Algren put it, "like a dying juke box in a deserted bar."

I remember my first glimpse of Cook County Hospital that morning. It was a chilly and gray day. The hospital was a Goliath that rose out of the West Side neighborhood just west of the Chicago Loop. Eight stories high, it loomed over Harrison Street below. Built in 1914 in the Beaux-Arts, neo-classical style popularized by the World's Columbian Exposition of 1893, it was long outdated. Patients were a secondary consideration from the start. The architect of the building was obsessed with creating a public monument and overran his budget, creating the now faded façade of columns, cornices and gargoyles whose yellow-brick face was darkened by years of soot and disrepair on its Harrison Street side. It looked sick and tired, grim and grimy. Not like any hospital I had seen before or since.

The hospital commanded an entire city block—Harrison on the north, Polk on the south, Wolcott on the west, and Wood on the east. Administrative buildings, the house staff living quarters and the large outpatient Fantus Clinic spilled over Wolcott Street towards Ogden Avenue. Pasteur Park, a postage stamp of green, fronting the hospital on its Harrison Street side, was dotted with a statue of French scientist Louis Pasteur, a few glum-looking trees, a heliport and a rundown Greek restaurant.

People loitered at the front entrance of the hospital smoking and chatting. Cars and buses rumbled down Harrison Street. A vendor hawked newspapers. A garbage can by the entrance overflowed with trash. Pieces of paper and assorted flotsam blew by. The two sets of double doors led into a marble-floored foyer, the floor darkened with gum splotches and grunge, while a Depression era, age-stained, eight-foot granite sculpture of a mother and children watched over the entrance. Another set of doors led to the dimly lit Harrison Street lobby with dark floors and vomit-green institutional glazed tile walls that reminded me of a post office or a train station waiting room. The sounds and smells in the lobby filled my senses. I was used to the clean antiseptic smell and the gleaming floors of a hospital. Not here. A tide of humanity stumbled and drifted in both directions down the hallway, a cacophonous amalgamation of sounds and voices. The lobby had a faint aroma of stale tobacco, musk, mildew and perspiration. The County Hospital lobby could have been mistaken for a Calcutta bus station, not a place of healing.

Dr. Quentin Young was a legend to us—a progressive doctor who had been, for the past six years, Chairman of the Department of Internal Medicine at Cook County. Dr. Young, Chicago-born and raised, had been an intern and resident at Cook County Hospital during its heyday from 1947 to 1952. In the 1950s and 1960s, Quentin made a name for himself as a young physician when he and others exposed the racist policies of Chicago hospitals that commonly excluded blacks from receiving care. He founded the Committee to End Discrimination whose aim it was to desegregate Chicago hospitals and medical organizations. This group reviewed the birth and death records at the Chicago Department of Health and found that blacks were born and usually died at only two hospitals in the city, Cook County and the black-owned Provident Hospital. This revelation and pressure from the federal government after the passage of Medicare began to open other institutions in Chicago to people of color.

Quentin was also known as a founder and past chairman of the Medical Committee for Human Rights—an organization of health care professionals who provided medical relief services during the civil rights and anti-war marches of the 1960s. We were familiar with Quentin and the Medical Committee for Human Rights from our readings in medical school. And Quentin had additional credentials to make him just the kind of role model we sought. He was a proponent of a national health service, a form of universal health coverage. He had been the personal physician for Martin Luther King Jr. when King moved to Chicago in 1966 to address the issue of racial discrimination in the north. And he was called before the House Committee on Un-American Activities to explain his role in the 1968 Democratic National Convention anti-war demonstrations in Chicago. During this testimony, Quentin cited his First Amendment right to speak and thus defended himself and others, making the committee, now in its final days, look foolish.

Quentin had accepted the position as Chairman of Medicine after the previous, popular Chairman was summarily fired by Dr. James Haughton, the Director of the Governing Commission. After the firing, the hospital spun out of control and many doctors left in protest. An activist member of the house staff told Dr. Haughton there was only one man who could "save his ass".... Dr. Quentin Young. Much to everyone's surprise, Quentin accepted the position.

Dr. Young's appointment caused consternation among some conservative members of the governing commission and some medical staff members aligned with the County Board. When one of the County Board Commissioners said that Dr. Young would get appointed, "over my dead body," Dr. Young, with characteristic good humor, responded, "It's a deal!"

Quentin inspired a renaissance of sorts at County. Many idealistic doctors had left County in the years before his arrival. His interest in the role of social conditions and deprivation on health attracted a new generation of attending and resident physician staff back to County Hospital. Another group of reinforcements had arrived at the front lines of the health care wars. Quentin's chairmanship was not without its challenges. After the House Staff strike at Cook County Hospital in 1975, Quentin was fired by the Governing Commission for siding with the young doctors. The House Staff took his office door off its hinges so management could not change the locks and held a twenty-four-hour vigil outside his office until he regained his position after a court fight. Today, in his late eighties, Quentin is still an activist and the nation's foremost proponent of a single-payer health care system.

We had arranged for Quentin to interview us as a group. Or, to be more precise, we arranged to interview Quentin. Group interviews for residency spots were uncommon, both then and now. The usual process is for a prospective resident to be invited in for an interview on a set day with other interviewees. Instead we invited ourselves.

Things went haywire as soon as we arrived at Quentin's office for the interview. We quickly learned that much about County Hospital was dysfunctional. We announced our presence to Quentin's secretary.

"What appointment?" she asked in her lilting Jamaican accent, looking at us with a bewildered expression. "You can't have an appointment with Dr. Young; he's out of town."

"Out of town?" I said. "How can he be out of town? We have traveled 800 miles to Chicago for an interview, and he's out of town!" I felt my temples tighten as if gripped by a vise. My pulse beat a drum-roll in my head. My mouth was cotton-ball dry. That fight or flight feeling rose into my chest. I was ready to flee. She shrugged and stared at us, as if this was usual operating procedure at County. And it was, as we soon learned.

Before we could get our bearings, one of our resident hosts whisked us out of the Department of Medicine offices and took us to a mass meeting being held by the unions in another building. Someone shoved a leaflet in my hand, which in bold letters shouted out the crisis. The Governing Commission was closing the psychiatric building and threatening closure of the whole hospital because of funding shortfalls. The meeting was an electric event. Speakers exhorted the excited crowd of house officers and hospital workers to protest the closings and warned that these cuts were the beginning of the closing of Cook County Hospital. Long-haired house-staff officers—mostly white and east Asian—were intermixed with the mostly black clerical workers, nurses and other hospital workers. The chairs in the room were nearly full. We found empty seats and tried to understand what was unfolding, while our minds were spinning and disoriented. One medical resident had heard we were prospective residency candidates here to interview. He leaned over, placed his hand on my shoulder in a reassuring gesture and said, "Ya gotta come here. It's great!"

Most medical students applying for a residency interview in a more formal manner. They don their dark suits and show up at the hospital for interviews, formal lunches and meetings with the faculty. They aim to train at academic medical centers, shining pinnacles of medical advancement. We, on the other hand, attended a mass meeting about the closing of the hospital after being stood up for our group interview.

By the end of the meeting I was sweaty and giddy with emotion, unable to sort out how I felt. But my body wasted no time weighing in. I felt a foul-tasting brash of acid in the back of my throat and a rumbling pressure in my lower abdomen that let me know I needed to find a toilet right away. I stumbled back to the main lobby through the swirl of people and tried to get the attention of the security guard at the front desk who was reading the *Sun-Times* as a beat-up black transistor radio played softly in the background.

"Can you tell me where the nearest bathroom is?" I asked, as the pressure on my sphincter reached the explosion point.

Without lifting his eyes from his paper he signaled with a finger to his left. There, in a nook at the side of the lobby, were the public toilets, men to the left and women to the right. In anticipation of immediate relief, I pushed open the grimy door, conscious of an oily film that stuck to my hands, the residue of thousands of Chicago hands.

It reeked. Clearly, it was not on the cleaning rotation. Stall doors were broken. Some were missing. Toilet seats were gone or broken, like the missing teeth of a skid row junkie. Brown, rust-tinged water filled the bowls. Urine deposits mottled the floors. There was no toilet paper. The row of white, chest-high urinals lined up like sentinels against the wall next to the sinks dripped water in a continuous hiss like an old steam radiator. I gagged. My intestines said yes; my nose and eyes said no. I twisted my intestines tight against the internal flood like the Dutch boy's finger in the dike, turned and ran back into the lobby.

The "Greeks" saved me. The "Greeks" was the greasy-spoon Greek restaurant across the street from County. I ran across Harrison Street, dodging traffic, and fast-walked into the Greeks. I was greeted by a white Formica diner counter with a display of pies and cakes in a glass carousel. A restaurant worker in a white cotton apron and cap stood behind the counter. He pointed me to the bathroom. Off to the right was a small room with booths. One wall was covered with paintings of monkeys. A bar lined another wall. Generations of County residents crossed Harrison Street to sit at a booth in the Monkey Room at the Greeks for a hamburger, fries or a beer during a night on-call, until the Greeks burned down in a mysterious fire a few years later.

I found my way to the bathroom. It was not much better than the one I had escaped at County, but time had run out. It would have to do. I held my breath, closed the flimsy metal lock on the stall door, and sat on the toilet. All around me were dirt-streaked, white plastic tiles covered with drawings and phone numbers.

"What am I getting myself into?" I thought. "Am I cut out for this?" The squalor of the hospital; the mass meeting; the threat that the hospital would close; the blown interview. Does coming here make sense? As my mind ruminated, my bowels expressed my doubts.

The next day, after a series of calls to the hospital by our resident friends, an interview was arranged with Dr. Young, who had returned to the hospital. We strode into his office, shook his hand, and sat down. His office was lined with bookshelves, from floor to ceiling. A large wooden conference table surrounded by assorted chairs stood off to the side. One window overlooking a roof or airshaft let little light into the office. Quentin's desk was covered with papers and open books. And Quentin ... he looked like an absent-minded college professor, his horn-rimmed glasses perched on his nose, a disheveled mop of salt and pepper hair and a quizzical expression. In his tweed sports jacket, he looked more like a favorite uncle at Sunday Brunch than a department chairman and radical physician.

This was not an interview, but an encounter session. Quentin spoke to us as if we were long-lost friends. He told how he felt beleaguered. He said that he came to County with the idea of attracting young physicians like us only to find himself at odds with the young radical physicians in his department—specifically Mardge, her husband Gordy and the other residents who were critical of his leadership. These were the same residents who were trying to recruit us to come. I felt like Dorothy when she discovered that the Wizard of Oz was just a country-potions salesman behind a curtain. Quentin, our hero, seemed so much larger in our readings than in this first meeting. We expected to be quizzed and interrogated to see if we were worthy enough to join County. We hoped to ask Quentin about his vision for the department and the hospital. In the end, it was more group therapy than interview. I think Quentin felt better than we did after the session. We thanked him and tramped out of his office more bewildered than exhilarated. By the end of the visit, we assumed that if we wanted to go to County, County would take us. And we hoped, but were not entirely confident, that the hospital would stay open.

Many years later my friend Steve Whitman told me of his interview with Quentin during the same period. Steve had been fired from his two prior teaching jobs because of his political views. In a desire to disclose his past fully, he told Quentin.

"I want you to know, I was fired from my last two jobs."

Quentin didn't miss a beat: "Oh, that's great," he said. "You'll fit right in here."

After the interview, we attended a morning report in Quentin's office—a session in which overnight admissions to the hospital were discussed. The cases involved clinical conditions that we had never seen in medical school. The level of the discussion was also impressive, and the residents and attending physicians were friendly and well-informed. After the morning report, we spoke with a number of house staff who all felt very happy to be training at Cook County Hospital. How exhilarating it was to have such a large group of opinionated, political, passionate young physicians in one place.

Clearly, Cook County Hospital was on the frontline battleground of the health-care crisis in America with lots of enemies who would have liked to see it closed. It was also decrepit, dysfunctional and depressing—a horrible place to treat patients. It was my first exposure to an institution that served mostly black people and I was shocked, but not surprised, by the abhorrent conditions. So by the end of a forty-eight-hour visit, despite moments of great apprehension and anxiety, my friends and I were ready to sign on the dotted line. And because we were American medical students, we knew we would be guaranteed spots in the training program that catered mostly to foreign-trained medical graduates. The five of us went back to Syracuse with our plans for residency set.

Residency selection in the U.S. was done by a computer, both then and now. Students have interviews in many places and then list their choices which are matched with the training programs' favorite candidates. It was a crap shoot. We knew it was unlikely that the computer would match a group of friends to train at the same place. We foiled the system. Cook County Hospital was the only institution we placed on our match lists. By only listing one institution we were guaranteed to continue our training together at County. Because our medical school experience had been so disappointing, we asked County if we could do part-time residency programs. Rather than work all year, we requested that four of us share three spots. We would be paid less and have an extra year of residency but we also would have four months off each year. They agreed. A fifth student applied to the Pediatric residency. Two others would follow us to Chicago the next year.

Immediately, the backlash began. When our professors at Syracuse heard we all planned to go to Cook County Hospital rather than an academic medical center, they tried to dissuade us. One professor told me that Cook County was about to be disaccredited and that working there was akin to working in a jungle—a response I rejected as racist. Many of our professors interpreted our decision as their failure. But we were hardheaded and disregarded every attempt to change our minds. I was reassured when my father, despite his reservations about my wounded pigeon tendencies, encouraged me to go.

Had we been able to Google at the time, we would have come across an article from July 1970 in the *Chicago Tribune Magazine* called, "The Trouble with County. Some folks say it rose up from hell. And to hell it almost returned." It portrayed the gritty politics of County Hospital in the late 1960s and presaged the battles that we would face a decade later. In the 1930s through the 1950s, County was one of the premier locations for residency training in the U.S. But years of near-criminal neglect had rendered it a training backwater, a place for misfits, idealists, foreign-trained doctors seeking an American toehold and radicals with visions of changing the world. While we felt like pioneers, full of energy and ready to confront the challenges of improving health care in Chicago, truth be told, we were more like reinforcements at battlefront trenches in a long, drawn-out war. We would be lucky not to experience the fate of a long line of idealistic physicians who came to Cook County Hospital before us, many of whom left cynical, demoralized and defeated. Corruption, race politics and political patronage had all but sucked the lifeblood from County Hospital in the years before we arrived. Had we really understood how bad things were, we might have reconsidered our decision. But we were not concerned with the risks and only saw the benefits of this decision. We were ready to cast our lot with County come hell or high water.

Match day is one of the high points of the U.S. medical school experience. This was the day when all prospective residents found out where they would be doing their residency training. Like the Oscars, envelopes were handed out and the applicants nervously fumbled to rip them open to see where the computer had matched them. Tears of joy and whoops filled the air. We skipped Match day. Our fates were in our own hands. Cook County Hospital. We'd fit right in.

CHAPTER 4

July 1978: Sink or Swim

I DID NOT LOOK LIKE A DOCTOR. Not in the traditional sense, at least. None of us did. My hair was long and in a tight, curled "afro." I sported a moustache that overhung my top lip. My sartorial style could best be classified as early twentieth-century mountain woodsman. I had a penchant for flannel shirts in the winter, short sleeves in the summer, corduroys, and earth shoes or Birkenstocks. A tie or white coat was out of the question. After three years of residency, the three white coats I was given during the first days of my internship remained in their original plastic bags, untouched.

In my preparation for internship, I went to an Army-Navy supply store and purchased an Army surplus knife sheath in camouflage green canvas, imprinted with "U.S." in bold black letters to hold my medical equipment. It had a loop that I attached to my belt. When I walked into County on July 1, 1978, I looked like a cross between Rambo and Doogie Howser. In truth, I was scared shitless about the prospects of starting internship. I rued all the lectures that I had skipped and the times I slacked off in medical school. I worried about whether I would be good enough. In truth, I was an average medical student, square in the middle of my class. There were whole categories of diseases that had just passed me by. As I stood on the precipice of my residency at Cook County, I gulped down my feelings of inadequacy. Inside, I was a quivering bag of nerves.

Our reputation preceded us. We were referred to as the "Syracuse group" to distinguish us from the "Rush Mafia"—a large group of residents, including Mardge Cohen, her husband Gordy Schiff, and others. They had come from Rush Medical College across the street. There was a group of black residents as well. Many were born and raised in Chicago, had trained in the Urban Health Program at the University of Illinois Medical School and viewed a residency at County as a way to serve their own communities. Most prominent and vocal among these black physicians was Cleveland-born Linda Rae Murray, at five foot two, a solidly built, militant health activist and gifted orator. She wore her hair in an afro, dark black with a streak of gray in the front, and carried herself with a self-confident swagger. She viewed us with skepticism. Chicago was her adopted home, the County patients her community. We were interlopers of sorts and new to Chicago. On the other hand, many of the black (and other) residents at County were there for the clinical experience and wanted nothing to do with the politics of the place. Linda was more akin to us in that way. Like us, she viewed her presence at County as part of a larger national struggle about race and health. In addition to the American residents, County had an equal number of foreign-trained (mostly Indian and Pakistani) physicians; for them, County was just like the institutions they had left back home—overcrowded, undersupplied, and decrepit. They were happy to have landed a training spot in the U.S. Many had already completed residencies back home in India and were more experienced than most of us.

July 1 was the start of internship at every hospital in the U.S. So it was for us. We sat in the large auditorium with over 100 interns from every medical and surgical discipline. The murmur of many separate conversations burbled through the air. As I scanned the room I saw a United Nations of young doctors representing many ethnicities, states and countries. Long hair and afros abounded. For the first time since starting medical school, I felt at home, despite the rumors about the hospital's persistent troubles. There was still talk about the hospital closing and layoffs of staff, but I was preoccupied with my own thoughts about not killing patients. I shoved my worries about the viability of the hospital to the recesses of my brain. There would be plenty of time to worry about that later. There was no turning back now. My career as a doctor was about to begin.

A stooped, elderly doctor in a starched white lab coat shuffled up to the podium. His face was lined and his dark bagged eyes under bushy salt-and-pepper eyebrows dissected the crowd. A hush came over the auditorium as he welcomed us in a guttural Eastern European accent that gurgled up from his throat, "Goot ahfterr-noon, dok-tors," he spoke with quivering jowls. "Vell-come, to Cook County Hospital." He was the famous Paul Szanto, a world-renowned pathol-ogist. He told us the story of how he had escaped from Hungary on the eve of World War II, one step ahead of the Nazis. Through some connections he landed a job at County. "Ven I got uff de ship in New York, in nineteen toity eight, my friends asked me where I vas goink to voik. I said, Cook County Hospital, Cheecago. They vere shocked and said to me, 'Dr. Szanto. Cook County Hospital? Ve hoid it vas closink!'" We laughed. A tension reliever. If in 1938 there were rumors of County closing we should not get overly concerned about the same rumors circulating in 1978, despite the dark rumblings on the horizon.

My first assignment was Ward 24, in the Main Hospital building. Ward 24 was the largest of the medical floors, located at the very end of the football-field-long central corridor on the far west side of the second floor of the main hospital. With the exception of a few two- and four-bed units, all patients were housed on this large open ward. It was about eighty feet long with fifteen or so hospital beds lined up side by side on either side of the room. Interspersed were large double-hung widows, their glass opaque with years of accumulated soot. County Hospital was not air-conditioned. My internship began in July, and the windows were cracked open, but the summer air hung still and stifling like a steam bath, blanketing the patients and staff. Large industrial fans were placed at the entrance to the floor in a futile attempt to move the air. Their roar made the ward sound more like a landing strip at Midway Field than a hospital. In those days patients were allowed to smoke on the floors, and the combination of smoke, body odor and illness contributed to the ambience.

Ward 24 was notorious for more reasons than its ambience and aroma. In 1956, an intern, Bruno Epstein, son of Jewish refugees from Austria, was murdered on Ward 24. In the 1950s there were no outpatient clinics and patients returned to the wards for their outpatient follow-up after surgery. The unsuspecting Bruno was confronted on the ward by a meat-cleaver-wielding Chinese patient who was unhappy with the results of his surgery a few weeks before. The patient stalked onto the floor determined to exact revenge. He did. Bruno was in the wrong place at the wrong time. The Chinese man cornered Bruno and yanked the cleaver from its hiding place in his pants. Screams and slashes ensued. Bruno staggered, mortally wounded, into the corridor and collapsed in a pool of blood as horrified interns and nurses looked on. A plaque memorializing Bruno Epstein and his untimely end was on the wall of the residents' lounge for all new interns to see. It said, "Died while serving the sick on Ward 24." The intern of the year award was named for poor Bruno. The irony of this inauspicious internship assignment on Ward 24, barely twenty years after Bruno's demise, did not escape me.

The assignment to Ward 24 was considered undesirable for more than Bruno's legacy. Some residents thought that the nurses on the unit were not as good as those on other units and that the patients were neglected. Actually, the nursing care left a lot to be desired throughout the institution. The nurses were short-staffed and poorly supervised. Like us. Especially late at night. Many nights I walked onto a darkened unit to treat a patient, and would need a nurse. There were none in sight. Patients moaned in their beds, unattended. I searched for help and found the nurses asleep in various nooks and crannies on the unit, covered in white flannel patient blankets on jerry-rigged chairs—one to sit on and another on which to rest their legs. This happened frequently enough to make me concerned about the quality of the nursing care.

Other residents complained that Ward 24 was too far away from Ward 35, the admitting ward in the Medical A Building. Because an intern was required to cover the sick patients on their home ward on admitting days, he or she needed to run back and forth from the Medical A Building where patients were admitted, to Ward 24 over a block away, many times during the day and night to attend to sick patients.

Shortly after my arrival, an enterprising resident created a short cut from the Medical A Building. This was one of many workarounds that people discovered to make work easier at County. He managed to open a fire door by Ward 23, the next ward over from Ward 24, and created a makeshift shim to keep it from locking again. This made it possible to shave off about five minutes in travel time between the two buildings. Rather than walk through the Emergency Department to the main lobby and then up the stairs to the second floor, one climbed on the external steel fire escape, rickety and rusty, behind the Emergency Department, up to the second floor roof area above, crossed the roof to the jerry-rigged fire door, and entered the middle of the second floor corridor of the main Hospital. During the summer months, one could enter Ward 23 directly, through an open screened window accessible from the roof, into the nurse's station, where they prepared medications. Suddenly Ward 24 was not so far off the beaten track. Generations of internal medicine residents used this shortcut, until it was discovered a decade later and closed down.

In 1978, open wards were unusual in American hospitals. Cook County Hospital, one of the oldest public hospitals in the U.S., was one of the last with open patient wards. It is hard to describe the indignity the patients experienced. The floor had a set of overhead lights. One switch turned all the lights on. So if a doctor was called in the middle of the night to evaluate a patient, when the lights were turned on, every patient except the deepest sleepers was awakened. The units offered no privacy. Each patient bed was separated from the other by cotton-polyester curtains. When a patient was experiencing Delirium Tremens and hallucinating or moaning in pain, everyone on the floor suffered as well. These open wards had been in continuous use since the hospital was built. And these same wards were occupied for more than twenty years after I completed my internship. If the hospital was not serving poor people and others who were deemed undesirable because of their alcoholism or drug use, housing patients on open wards might not have been tolerated for so long. It was hard not to be upset at the conditions.

One could easily access the floor from the street, so it was not unusual for heroin addicts who were in the hospital receiving intravenous antibiotics to climb down the stairwell and open the door for a drug-dealing friend with heroin to inject into their intravenous lines as a way to stave off withdrawal. It was also not uncommon to find an amorous couple, having met in the hospital, in bed together behind the curtains. Of course, the patients in the adjoining beds were unwilling voyeurs to these trysts.

As unbearable as the heat and humidity was in the summer, the cold in the open wards in the winter was worse. County had only two temperatures—too hot or too cold. In winter, the windows iced up and rattled in the Chicago wind. Patients shivered under thin blankets, and their attempts to get more blankets from administration fell on deaf ears, usually because there were too few supplies. Families often brought in blankets from home to keep their relatives warm. During my first summer of 1978, Chicago experienced a heat emergency, and a number of elderly patients from area nursing homes were brought to Cook County with heat stroke, only to be placed on sweltering floors where the ambient temperature was over 100 degrees.

Patients suffered other indignities beyond the heat and cold. There were daily shortages of soap, towels, toothbrushes, sheets and other simple amenities. The nursing staff, often overwhelmed with the patient load, could not or would not respond to simple needs. There was no functional nurse-call system by which a patient could get help. If a patient needed assistance he or she had to yell. On every floor, patients lay in beds and called out over and over, "Nurse . . .

Nurse . . . Nurse," like a skip in a record, until somebody came, or the patient gave up. Often, it was the latter.

The open wards had one men's bathroom, one women's bathroom and one shower room, located in the hallway between the hospital lobby and the open ward—a half block away from the beds. Many patients could not negotiate the distance and soiled themselves in bed. It was even farther to get to one of the two or three pay phones that rang all day long, waiting for someone to pick them up. As interns we learned not to answer them because if we did, we had to go find the patient the caller wanted to speak to, and we did not have the time. The horror of the conditions affected the staff in different ways. Some doctors and nurses became jaded and cynical. Others left after a year or two. Others, like me and my friends, got angry and redoubled our efforts.

County was a petri dish for vermin. The rats and cockroaches had free rein, and fruit flies hovered above the patients' beds on the wards. I had one patient in that first year who was recovering from Delirium Tremens, the hallucinations caused by alcohol withdrawal. I asked him to report to me if he had any more visual hallucinations so I could adjust his medication. On my morning rounds, he beckoned me over with his finger.

"Hey Doc," he said, "last night I thought I saw two large rats across the ward. Can ya give me more medication?"

After I examined him and spoke with other patients, I realized that these were not hallucinations. He really did see rats. I reassured him and went on with my work.

A doctor friend, Julio, told me about his first day as a medical student on the surgery service in the County Operating Rooms on the 7th floor of the Main Building. Their north-facing windows were open to allow air in.

"Where's the medical student?" the chief resident asked.

Julio had scrubbed his hands for ten minutes in the prescribed manner, supervised in exquisite detail by the attending physician, then donned his sterile gown and gloves. It was his first operation and he was eager to contribute. He stepped forward anticipating the opportunity to hold a scalpel or to suture.

"I'm Julio. The third year."

The chief resident looked him over from head to toe.

"See that fly over there?" Julio nodded and eyed a fly buzzing around the room. "Your job is to keep it away from the surgical site."

Julio chased the fly around for the duration of the operation.

Our on-call rooms, where we slept when we had a chance, were infested with roaches of all sizes. One rule every intern learned was never to put on a shoe without first checking for cockroaches. My routine went like this: if I received a page from my call room, I stomped my feet on the floor to get the roaches scurrying and then quickly put on my shoes. These conditions would be fodder for front-page news in the *Chicago Tribune* if they were discovered at a private hospital. At County, this was business as usual, expected, accepted and ignored. It seemed to us that no one really cared how poor patients were treated. On the contrary, the *Chicago Tribune,* the conservative paper that dominated Chicago news, never seemed to want to see improvements in care at County. They just wanted it closed. The sooner the better.

This was the environment I encountered during my first days of internship. My skills were limited. I was overwhelmed by the conditions—by the hurdles to good patient care and the sickness and neglect I saw. As an intern, I was thrown in. It was sink or swim. I did a little of both.

CHAPTER 5

1978: The Cure

COUNTY WAS DESIGNED FOR FAILURE. The long distances between the floors made patient care difficult. But there was one place that was brilliant in its design, at least for green interns like me. The admitting unit, Ward 35. In most hospitals, sick patients are admitted to the next available bed and the physician and nurse go to that unit to administer treatment. At County, all patients came to one floor, Ward 35, to be evaluated or "worked up" as we call it. On a routine admission day at Cook County Hospital in 1978, forty to sixty patients were admitted over a 24-hour period and their care divided among the on-call residents.

While medical school covered the basics, I had big gaps in my knowledge and experience. These were the sickest patients I had ever seen. There was so much I did not know. And at County that was not an excuse. It was simple—you either performed or patients would die. The training wheels were off. But on Ward 35 all the residents and interns were together for a 24-hour period and we all learned from each other. If one person did not know the answer, someone else did. The collective wisdom and camaraderie of the doctors and nurses on Ward 35 added a level of security to what could otherwise be a terrifying experience.

Ward 35 was located in the Medical A Building on the third floor, the "newest" building on the County campus, built in 1925. It was an open ward with space for about twenty stretchers. Curtains separated each stall. At one end of the ward were two desks, back to back, where nurses and doctors sat to write their notes and look out over all the patients. At the other end of the room was a small metal table with four or six chairs where residents kept their supplies. Beyond the table there was a fire-escape door. The door was kept open in summer to let air in. Sometimes the residents and nurses sat out on the exposed steel fire escape to catch a break from the chaos.

Admissions rolled in from the Emergency Room, one after another, on stretchers or in wheelchairs. Patients who had already been worked up were moving in the other direction, to fill beds on the home wards scattered around the hospital grounds. It was a delicate balance, and when the incoming patients arrived more quickly than the outgoing could be cleared out, patients were lined up in rows, up and down the middle of the room. We called this a "middle row." It was not unusual, late on an admission night, for the metal table by the fire escape to have residents sitting next to patients in their wooden wheel chairs, waiting. Sometimes, for some patients, a stretcher never became available, and we were forced to interview and examine them in full view of everyone in the room—doctors, nurses, and other patients. It violated our beliefs about patient rights, but the conditions obliged us to act against our best intentions.

Ward 35 was a raucous and unruly floor. Patients screamed in pain and distress.

"Help me, Jesus! Help me, Jesus! Help me, Jesus!" they yelled.

The nurses were often too overwhelmed to respond immediately and shouted for assistance. Interns interviewed patients with voices raised in order to be heard above the din. Residents demanded charts. The overhead PA squawked when admissions arrived on the floor. Patients in Delerium Tremens hallucinated and clamored to be released from their full leather restraints. All the while, X-ray technicians circulated, flashed portable chest X-rays on patient after patient, while everyone in the room was exposed to radiation. They shouted, "X-Ray," and if we heard them, we all took a few steps back and then resumed our activities. How far back did we step? To this day, I have no idea. We were never instructed. There was nothing in the design of the room to shield us from the deadly X-rays. Twenty years after my residency, I developed a type of thyroid cancer linked to radiation exposure, which I attributed to my time on Ward 35.

My first patient at Cook County was an elderly African American woman, admitted with a failing heart. She sat up on the gurney that brought her from the Emergency Room, her gray wig askew, her face crisscrossed with wrinkles and her cheeks puffing in and out like bellows as she fought to get air. One leg dangled, swinging back and forth off the side of the cart, swollen with retained fluid, a characteristic of this condition. She leaned forward with both arms extended, her hands on her knees as she struggled to catch her breath. Her lungs were filling with fluid and she needed immediate treatment. A clear, green plastic tube which ended in a harness around her head delivered oxygen to her nose from a large steel oxygen tank next to her bed. I summoned up my bravado and approached her bed; my canvas army surplus holster slapped my thigh. With a tentative grin I introduced myself as her doctor, suddenly self-conscious about my appearance. She eyed me with suspicion, a look of skepticism and fear. She turned to her nurse, a large-boned, no-nonsense black woman packed into a starched white nurse's uniform, a size or two too small. As the patient gasped between breaths she said, "I ... ain't ... gonna ... let that little white boy ... woik on me!" I stopped, speechless. I threw a lost puppy gaze to the nurse who rolled her eyes at me.

The irony of the moment hit me at once. I had come to County to be together with my friends, to join other health activists, to work part time, to join the union, to fight racism, to improve health care for poor people and to learn medicine. Grand plans. Summarily rejected by a grandmother on a gurney on Ward 35. This "little white boy" was teetering on the edge. The nurse, whose jaundiced eyes had seen plenty of greenhorns like me pass through, jumped to my rescue and convinced the patient that despite my youthful and disheveled appearance, I was indeed a doctor. Where was my white coat when I needed it? This episode was a reality check and made me realize that if I did one thing during my time here, it would be to learn to be the best possible doctor for my patients.

One of the worst things to happen on-call was admitting a patient who needed a brain scan. County Hospital had no CAT scanners, which are special X-ray machines used to do brain scans. Patients who needed CAT scans had to be transferred to Presbyterian hospital—the private hospital across the street—accompanied by an intern. This whole process could take about four hours and set you back the whole night because the admissions did not stop while you were away. Adding insult to injury, the hapless intern needed to bring all kinds of medication across the street with him or her. If for some reason the patient had a cardiac arrest at Pres, the intern had to resuscitate the patient alone and needed to be well supplied. We had been told that Pres residents were not going to help if a patient arrested.

One patient still haunts me. A young man about 26 years old who was brought to the hospital in a confused state. There was disagreement about the cause. One doctor thought his condition was from drug use. I thought he might have head trauma or meningitis, both potentially more serious conditions. If we'd had a CAT scanner on site, we could have solved the dilemma quickly. A CAT scan at Presbyterian would take hours, which was too long. When he spiked a fever, my suspicion of meningitis increased, and after consulting with the other residents, I decided to perform a spinal tap. A small needle is placed in the spinal canal. Spinal fluid is drawn off and examined through a microscope. If an infection is present, high dose antibiotics are given. A simple procedure. But, a spinal tap without a brain scan was risky at times. If he had any brain swelling, common after head trauma, removing spinal fluid to look for meningitis might cause his brain to herniate—to be sucked down the spinal canal and crushed— a potentially fatal complication.

I prepared the spinal tap. A group of residents and interns stopped what they were doing and gathered around the patient's bed. One doctor stood on one side of the gurney and squeezed the patient's head and knees in a bear hug, forcing the patient into the fetal position and exposing his spinal column. I was on the other side of the gurney. The spinal kit was on a stand near the stretcher. I cleaned off the spot on his spine with iodine and inserted the needle into the spinal canal. I felt the pop as the needle passed into the spinal canal, and a jet of spinal fluid shot out. High pressure. Oh shit. I yanked the needle out as fast as I could to minimize the damage. Too late. The damage was done. High pressure spinal fluid meant brain swelling. Shortly thereafter, one of his pupils became dilated, a sign that his brain was beginning to herniate down his spinal canal. I called the neurosurgery residents who came to the bedside and drilled two burr holes in his skull to try to relieve the pressure on his brain. All because we had no CAT scanner. The patient survived, but suffered permanent brain damage.

We were practicing Third World medicine in Chicago, one of the largest cities in the U.S. I shudder to think how many patients I may have harmed or killed because we could not diagnose or treat them quickly enough—and this, because they were County patients and lacked access to the most basic services. It was battlefield medicine and I was forced to learn from my mistakes and move on.

One night on Ward 35 the admissions were rolling in. The middle row was stuffed with wheelchairs and stretchers. I had already admitted six or seven patients and was hours behind schedule. The overhead speaker squawked, "Admission!" Uh oh. I was summoned to the clerk's office to get the Emergency room chart. This was an elderly Chinese immigrant who spoke no English. To make matters worse, he was also deaf.

One thing you learned early on at County was the pecking order in the institution. In the late seventies, the attending physicians were somewhere at the bottom of that order; the resident physicians were somewhat higher. At the top of that pecking order were the ward clerks. They ran the hospital. Nothing got done at County without the acquiescence of the ward clerks. Most of them were streetwise, jaundiced black women who lived in the South and West Side ghettos of Chicago. You could not put anything past them. They had seen generations of young doctors come through County, each cohort with their lofty dreams and aspirations who had to confront the hard realities of County Hospital. The ward clerks were the unofficial den mothers to each new batch of interns, dishing out tough love and advice. Part drill sergeant and part wise auntie, you crossed them at your peril. They could and would make your work life unbearable. If you were rude or disrespectful to them, watch out. You would pay the price. Most savvy interns learned this lesson early.

Reba Maclin was the night admitting clerk on Ward 35, and she determined the admission assignments. Round but solidly built with obsidian skin and almond eyes, her hooded eyelids were highlighted with light blue eye shadow. She was a no-nonsense woman in her mid-thirties. She dominated the admitting ward like a barnyard dog. She had a razor-sharp tongue that kept interns in place but a big smile as well that she revealed if you earned it. You couldn't think of coming into her office copping an attitude. She cut through you like a buzz saw.

But that night, I was at my wit's end and knew I had to take her on. She assigned me the deaf Chinese man when I was already overwhelmed with sick patients. If I had to take this new patient, I did not think I could make it through the night. It wasn't that I minded taking patients, but I had to be able to talk to them.

I cautiously approached Reba's desk, perspiration beading on my brow, as much out of intimidation as from the humidity in the breezeless office.

"What do you want, Dr. Ansell?" she asked. "I just gave you a patient."

"Uh, uh, uh," I stammered. "Ms. Maclin, could you please assign me a different patient? Because this ..."

From her perch behind the desk, she scowled. Then let loose:

"You can kiss me all over and call me shorty, Ansell," she said. "Don't be coming into my office and tell me how to do my business."

I shrank, mumbled a hasty apology, and skulked out of the room. The last thing I wanted to do was to get on Reba's bad side. Lucky for me, I caught a break. One intern on-call that night was Alton Wong, a Chinese-American. I convinced him to trade patients with me, and he took the history from the deaf Chinese man in written Mandarin. The deaf man sat in his wooden wheelchair, in the middle of the open ward packed with patients, oblivious to the din, as he exchanged Chinese glyphs in silent dialogue with Dr. Wong.

As a young doctor from a small upstate New York town, I was exposed to a side of life I could never have experienced otherwise. I learned a lot about the strength and resolve that our patients and their families had, despite a society and health-care system that seemed to be stacked against them. And I learned about the dark side of life in Chicago. I learned the intricacies of drug use from patients, from the amount of heroin in a $10 bag to skin-popping Ts and Blues for a cheap high. I learned about Chicago history from pimps, drug dealers, and winos. One such patient had been a desk clerk at one of the notorious flop houses on Chicago's West Side "Skid Row," where hundreds of transient men and women had lived and died since the early 1900s. He described to me how, as a Democratic precinct captain in the 1960 presidential election, he had a few of his resident winos vote repeatedly, using the names of everyone who was ever listed in his flophouse guestbook. They did so gladly in exchange for shots of whiskey. So there was truth to the old Chicago adage, "Vote early, vote often!"

I also learned about street life in Chicago. One night a young kid arrived on Ward 35, found on the street, agitated and unresponsive, having overdosed on "Angel Dust," a commonly-abused horse tranquilizer. We tied him down in full leather restraints on a gurney as the drug wore off. I went through his moneyless wallet and found a phone number of a family member. Thirty minutes later, the kid's big brother, a muscle-bound street tough, swaggered in, his neck-breaking longshoreman arms bulging through his leather jacket, a Marlboro tucked behind his ear. He seemed less interested in his brother's condition than whether his money had been stolen.

"Did he have any money?" the tough guy asked.

"Nope," I replied. "His wallet was empty."

"Shii . . . t," he said, as he dragged out the curse like the fading whistle of a passing train, shaking his head in disgust. "I told the little punk not to keep his money in his wallet." He circled his brother's gurney with a scowl of disgust on his face, then stalked off the unit.

When little brother awoke the next morning, I informed him that he had no money in his wallet and had probably been robbed. He grinned and pried into his right sock to reveal a stashed wad of bills. "I never keep my money in my wallet. My brother taught me to keep it in my socks." Touché.

We had a small laboratory off Ward 35 where we learned to stain body fluids with Acid Fast to diagnose tuberculosis and Gram's stain to diagnose other bacterial infections. The instructions were on the wall behind the sink. The learning methodology at County was "see one, do one, teach one," and after a brief orientation by a senior resident to the glories of staining specimens, I was on my own. Taped on the wall of this makeshift laboratory by an enterprising resident at one point during my residency were the words of Rudyard Kipling's poem "If." In my own head I rewrote Kipling's poem: If we could somehow survive this, if we could get through one more hot summer's night, through this year, then maybe we would all be men and women. We sat at the table in the laboratory, our fingertips stained with blue, red, and purple, as if at a psychedelic finger-painting party, and peered into our microscopes attempting to make diagnoses. If something unusual was present, all fourteen residents and myriad students gathered to take a look.

When a patient went into cardiac arrest, as often happened in those days, someone yelled "Code!" and we all dropped whatever we were doing and ran to help our colleagues revive the patient. The other patients in the room gawked, helpless and frightened observers in gurneys and wheelchairs, as we attempted to save a life. Many a night, I sat by the bedside of a sick asthmatic, his or her rapid wheezes and air hunger a sign of respiratory collapse. I tried to nurse them through the night, administering medication and encouragement to keep them off the ventilator.

Every so often Ward 35 settled down into a manageable chaos, and my co-interns and I sat and talked through the night about our aspirations, our families, our politics and our dreams for the future, as if we were sitting at a coffeehouse, not in a public hospital admitting floor.

My friends from medical school and I were assigned to different admitting services and we saw each other only in passing on the wards, in the cafeteria or at demonstrations downtown. County was such a big place I sometimes went days without seeing any of them. They each had their own admitting-floor experiences, and it was not too long before our skills improved and we all felt more comfortable in our roles as doctors. The anxiety attacks that began in medical school stopped. Cold. My medical school colleague with the rashes? Cured. And my other friend, Jim Schlosser, said, "I got an ulcer in medical school and it went away during internship."

CHAPTER 6

1978: Is There a Doctor in the House?

I WAS IN OVER MY HEAD. I made mistakes. I did not know enough. What's worse, my ignorance harmed patients. County was a resident-run hospital, a classic case of the inmates running the asylum. We residents and our patients suffered from not having the most expert doctors help make day-to-day decisions. It was only years later, when I became an attending physician, that I realized what a deficit we faced.

Late one afternoon I was called by another resident to see a patient who had lingered on the orthopedic floor for days with a serious infection of his leg. I came to see him at 6:00 p.m. after a long workday. I was exhausted and wanted to get home. I shuffled to the patient's bedside at the end of the ward. The patient was a toothless middle-aged man who lived in a flophouse on Chicago's Skid Row. He was delirious with fever and writhed back and forth in pain. His leg was swollen, red and angry, hot with infection. I agreed to have him transferred to the medicine service. It never crossed my mind to discuss it with the attending physician whose name was on the consult schedule with me. It just was not done. I failed to understand how serious and deep the infection was—he had a flesh-eating infection that a more experienced physician might have recognized. The next day I found the patient. On a ventilator. In the intensive care unit. An infectious disease specialist examined him and criticized me for not recognizing this deadly disease. The patient required emergency surgery. Too little, too late. He died.

People died because County lacked equipment. People died because of delays. Sometimes, people died because of our inexperience. Pick your poison. We had too few ICU beds to manage all the patients who were critically ill, so we managed them on the wards. Our nurses were overworked and harassed. Medicines did not always come up from the pharmacy. Crucial tests like X-rays were delayed or not done.

The same was true on the surgery side of the house. Residents in surgery were sometimes left to do operations on their own without an attending physician in the hospital. At times the attending was not in the country. Nowadays this would almost never happen. But then, by the time the surgeons hit their third year they had done hundreds of operations, many of them on their own. In the end they became excellent surgeons, but their learning was at the expense of the patients. Our patients deserved better. It was an issue of equity and fairness. The training experience was not for the weak-kneed or faint of heart. We were "doctors within borders," often the last hope for our patients. Sometimes we eked out a save. Made a great diagnosis. Sometimes we came up short for our patients. The best of us learned to think on our feet and get better. We taught each other. Shared articles and pointers. I spent the better part of my internship in pursuit of other residents for advice. The worst of us were hopelessly lost because of our lack of knowledge and guidance. This is not to say that there were no experienced physicians around. There were some attending physicians but they were disengaged from the day-to-day issues of patient care, and never available at night or on weekends. I had one attending who rounded with us in the cafeteria. He never saw a patient in the hospital.

Sometimes the cycle-time between learning and doing was a little too close for comfort. One day I heard an attending cardiologist talk about the physical findings we should look for when a patient had a serious form of a punctured and collapsed lung—a sound called a "Hamman's crunch," caused by the heart lining smacking against the lining of a collapsed left lung. I had never heard of it before and filed it away. A few nights later, at 3:00 a.m., I was called to the trauma unit at the request of a surgery resident. There, on the examination table was a middle-aged man, extremely short of breath, leaning forward on his arms, gasping for air. From his looks, his barrel chest and the nicotine stains on his fingernails, he was what we call a "big time smoker" and probably had severe emphysema.

The trauma unit was a room on the third floor of the main hospital. Because it was the middle of the night, all the lights were off except for those illuminating the patient. It was very quiet and except for the surgery resident, the gasping patient and me, no one else was around.

"What's up?" I asked the surgery resident. He glanced over at me, a tight-lipped grimace on his face. He was clearly nervous.

"This guy fell and broke a rib. He has asthma. Can you tell me what dose of asthma meds I should give him?" I was an expert in asthma by now and could rattle off the treatments for asthma in my sleep. But I was suspicious.

"Sure," I said, "but let me examine him first." I eyed the patient. He was struggling for air. I could see his ribs and neck muscles strain with each breath, a sign of failing lungs. In addition to his rapid breathing, his heart was racing. Not good. I listened to his lungs and I did not hear any breath sounds over his left lung, the side of the fractured rib. As I listened more closely, I heard a clicking sound with every rapid breath—could this be Hamman's crunch—the sign of a collapsed lung? On the right side he had some air flow but no wheezes. Asthma was not the cause of his shortness of breath.

"Did you treat him with anything?" I asked the surgeon.
"Yeah, I gave him an inter-costal block to blunt the pain of the fracture."

An inter-costal block is a dose of local anesthetic given to the nerve that runs between the ribs. It is used sometimes to blunt the pain from a rib fracture. Sometimes the needle used to give a nerve block can accidentally puncture the lung and cause it to collapse. In a guy like this with bad lungs to begin with, it can be deadly.

"Do you have a chest X-ray?" I asked. The resident pointed out the chest X-ray on a viewing monitor across the room. The light from the viewing monitor lit up the otherwise dark corner of the room with a bright fluorescent glow. The X-ray exhibited the typical findings one would expect in a man with severe emphysema. The lungs were over-expanded and the diaphragms were flattened out. This guy must have smoked more than the Marlboro Man. I did not see any sign of lung collapse on this X-ray. As my eyes passed back and forth between the X-ray and the struggling patient on the table, I was disturbed about this discrepancy between my exam and the X-ray. I listened to the patient's chest again and heard the crunch of his heart smacking the collapsed lining of his left lung. No time for waffling, I had to make a call.

"Put a needle in his chest!" I said to the surgeon, my voice rising, "He doesn't need treatment for asthma; he has a tension pneumothorax!"

A tension pneumothorax is a condition where the air escapes from the lung usually from an accidental perforation and gets caught between the chest wall and the lung, causing the lung to collapse. If not treated, the patient will die. This can be caused by a rib fracture or a stick by a needle. The treatment is simple and drastic. Time is of the essence. A needle is inserted into the chest to let the air out—like a valve on a tire. This man was on the verge of collapsing. Hamman's crunch was the clue.

"But the chest X-ray is normal. He can't have a pneumothorax," the surgeon protested. He was right. If a patient had a pneumothorax, the collapsed lung would be seen on X-ray. But this X-ray had been taken hours before, in the emergency room. Despite County having the finest trauma unit in the city and perhaps the country, it was the middle of the night. It could take hours to get someone up from the Radiology Department to repeat the film. If we had repeated it immediately, it might have confirmed my clinical hunch and allowed the surgeon to proceed with more confidence. But this was County, and sometimes we had to wing it.

The young surgeon gulped. He was no older than I. Two rookies. We had never met before. Could he trust me? Probably, he had never done this procedure. Neither had I. The patient's staccato breathing was the only sound in the room. The surgeon grabbed a needle and a syringe, with reluctance. He looked over at me, eyebrows raised, as if to say, "Here goes nothing." It was late. We both had been up since early morning the day before. No one else was around. Our backs were against the wall. The patient would likely die if we did not act. I held my breath as he pushed the needle into the chest wall of the gasping patient.

"Hissssssssssss!" The trapped air fizzled from the chest cavity like a balloon sputtering air, and the patient's breathing settled down. A save. Lucky this time. It could have gone the other way.

That's what County was like—sometimes glory and sometimes defeat. The stress of working under these conditions got to all of us after a while. We all broke. I was told that once J. W., a tough New York woman, wild-eyed and high-strung, a few years ahead of me in residency, stood outside the A Building and smashed empty glass blood vials one after another against the outside brick wall in silent rage. On another occasion, she got into a fist fight with a clerk who would not hand over an X-ray. I reached my own breaking point about two months into my internship year.

Sleeplessness and the patient load wore me down. What drove me mad was the re-work. The patients did not get their X-rays. They had to be re-ordered. The medications were not given. I had to check each one. The patients did not get transported for tests. It gnawed at me. I was working 100 or more hours a week. Punch drunk from sleep deprivation.

I finally lost it. My tipping point. Over a missed blood draw. A small thing. It happened every day at County. A snafu. Situation normal, all fucked up. But this particular day. I decided that once and for all, I was going to get to the bottom of this incompetency—AND FIX IT!

There was only one official blood-draw daily. This "perk" was part of the contract that was negotiated after the House Staff strike three years before. But there was a catch. The intern placed the lab requests in a folder for the clerk the evening before. If the unit clerk on the floor failed to post the blood-draw requests in time, the laboratory staff would not draw the blood. The intern then had to walk to the floor, draw and label all the patients' blood work for the day. It was the bane of an intern's existence and took hours out of the day. Scut work. So the last thing I did before I transferred a patient from the admitting ward to the home ward was to write down all the laboratory orders that needed to be drawn the next day.

One post-call day, hectic and harried, I arrived on Ward 23 to find that the orders I had so meticulously written out had not been executed. I had to traipse the length of the unit and perform all the daily draws myself. I seethed with each draw. I was tired. Cranky. I wanted revenge. Justice would be served! I surmised that the culprit must have been the evening clerk, Mrs. Jones, and decided to confront her when she arrived at three. I staked out my position near the clerk's station on Ward 23 and waited. My mouth tasted like cheap machine coffee. My armpits were sweaty from sleep deprivation and my face and forehead had a greasy sheen. I had not slept in thirty-six hours.

I watched as Mrs. Jones strolled onto the ward. She was a large-boned woman with a round, full-cheeked face, reddened with just a little too much blush. She wore a dress and high heels under her open white coat. Her hair had been relaxed and hair-sprayed into a beehive shape, lacquered high and thick atop her head like a rain-darkened cumulus cloud. Her nails, long and curled, were painted cherry red. She carried a copy of the New Testament in her hand. Its brown cover, with gold inlay lettering worn from years of handling. A staff nurse greeted her,

"Good afternoon, Mrs. Jones. How are you today?"

"Blessed," Mrs. Jones replied.

Blessed? Blessed? I waited until she was seated. I watched as she squeezed herself into the desk chair which just accommodated her full figure. She placed her Bible on the desk next to the phone, careful to make sure it was within reach. Her black mascara-enhanced brown eyes sparkled under the fluorescent lights as she surveyed her work station with pride and made a few last touches, like an actress about to take the stage. The Bible was moved a little closer. She smiled in satisfaction and placed her hands in front of her on the table. I pounced.

"Mrs. Jones?" I enquired. I forced a grin which felt more like a grimace.

"Yes, Dr. Ansell? Good afternoon," she responded, with a wide, gap-toothed smile. I launched in. I told her about all my patients who had been sent over and the fact that none of their labs had been taken off. I raged about how hard this had made the day for me. When I came up for air, she responded.

"I don't know what you are talking about, Dr. Ansell, I took all the labs off." I was hoping for a simple apology. All she had to do was admit it! I was not prepared for an outright denial. I snapped. "No you didn't. You're lying," I blurted, as my voice rose in pitch, like a kettle about to boil. A plume of anger rose from the pit of my stomach, a volcanic stream of red-hot magma suddenly released after weeks of unrelenting frustration, sleeplessness, indignities, and the stress of internship at County. I felt it rise to my chest and throat. My clenched teeth ached and the backs of my eyes began to burn as I struggled to keep from exploding in molten fury. But it was too late. I spewed. A burst of invective and curses followed: "I am tired of this fucking, goddamn, bullshit that goes on all the time around here...." my voice became louder and louder as both hands gesticulated wildly with each wave of this diatribe. I attracted a crowd of residents and nurses, their heads peeked in and out of the clerk's office, like prairie dogs at a coyote sighting. My tirade trailed off as quickly as it began. My shoulders slumped. I was spent, exhausted and depleted. All activity on the unit had come to a standstill.

Mrs. Jones sat. Silent. Serene. Not a sprayed hair out of place. Her chunky hands were clasped like a schoolgirl, in front of her on the desk. Her eyes blinked in rapid succession, the only sign of emotion. I stared, my eyes bulging, as I waited for her rebuttal. "Bring it on, Mrs. Jones. Bring it on," I thought.

After a very long while, during which her eyes held my gaze, she spoke. "Dr. Ansell," she cooed in a voice of treacle with a trace of a Southern accent. She paused for a second or two before continuing, "Please don't speak to me like that. Don't you know that I am a lady?"

"Oh, Oh . . . A lady," I repeated to myself. I was stopped in my tracks. The case had been prosecuted in my head over and over. Now the jury had spoken: "A lady." Suddenly, the crime of the missing labs was not a big deal. My behavior was. I had just spouted like a drunken sailor to a . . . "lady." I felt sick. I needed a different strategy if I was going to survive County. I sighed, apologized to Mrs. Jones, and slinked away.

I discovered a new way to manage stress during that first dark winter of internship. After a long day of work, my friend Stuart Kiken and I zipped into hooded sweatshirts, put on sweatpants, shoved our work clothes into our Jansports and rode the evening commuter el from the Polk Street Station near County to Randolph and Michigan. We did not get out of work until 6:00 or 7:00 p.m. and the train was stuffed with work-weary commuters wrapped thick in winter clothes. My mind was numbed after a full day at the hospital and I unwound as the train rumbled and shook from stop to stop on its way to the Loop. I'd make mental lists of my patients and what I had to do. Stuart and I barely spoke as we held the straps and transitioned from the hospital back to our civilian lives. The wind whipped south down Michigan Avenue, whistled against the high-rises and slapped the exposed parts of our faces. The dark of the cold winter's night contrasted with the bright lights of the Magnificent Mile. We ran north, heads down against the screeching wind, past shop windows, hotels and straggling shoppers, five or six miles through Lincoln Park to our apartments in Wrigleyville. When we reached the snow-blanketed solitude of Lincoln Park, we had a ritual. I signaled my pal with a raised finger.

"Get ready, one . . . two . . . three!" and at the count of three Stuart and I screamed at the top of our lungs until they were depleted of air and our vocal cords were raw.

Our blood-curdling screeches fractured the Arctic silence of Lincoln Park and were muffled by the snow drifts and the swirling wind. We howled for the indignities our patients faced. We howled for the lack of support services at the hospital. We howled for our inexperience and frustrations. We howled for the patients who died on our watch. When the gut-wrenching last wail dissipated into the chill of the night we laughed at the absurdity of our situation until tears rolled down our cheeks. Both the running and the screaming must have helped because I bounced out of bed the next day, raring to go at it again.

CHAPTER 7

General Medicine Clinic

AUGUST, 1978. DOG DAYS IN CHICAGO. The windows overlooking Ogden Avenue were open in a futile attempt to induce a breeze. A kamikaze fly buzzed my head. The air was thick as syrup. My shirt was Saran Wrap plastered to my body. A distant rumble from trucks and cars that barreled past the clinic on Ogden waltzed its way up the four floors to the cubicle where I sat. The room was no larger than a closet. A chair and an examination table wedged in. No sink. A partition about seven feet high separated my stall from the next one. A polyester curtain provided a flimsy barrier between the exam room and peeping eyes from the hall outside. A pile of dog-eared manila folders and blank yellow-lined progress notes that passed for patient charts were stacked on the desk in front of me.

During the three years of residency, each internal medicine resident was assigned a half-day every week in the clinic. Interns were thrown in every August, just handed a schedule and told to show up. After a month on the County wards you were deemed ready to tackle outpatient medicine. I was led to my cubicle by a hard-nosed clinic nurse. Part clinician and part traffic cop, these nurses ran the clinics. The waiting area resembled Union Station, with back-to-back, church-pew-like benches, lined end-to-end down the center of the hallway. Stuffed with patients. Their eyes followed me as I passed by.

Technically, we were supervised by an attending physician. Mine was a well-known schmoozer. From my cubicle I could look down the hall to the office where he was ensconced like a night watch-man, the door ajar, his legs on the desk and a phone receiver wedged between his shoulder and his ear. A sweet arrangement. We ignored him. He ignored us. Voices carried from cubicle to cubicle. No privacy. I learned outpatient medicine by eavesdropping on the conversations that other young doctors in the stalls around me had with their patients.

In the midst of the politics, the chaos, the poor physical condition of County Hospital, the hard, urban rudeness of the clerks and other staff, my clinic cubicle would become a place of refuge for me. I was home. It was my calling to be a primary care doctor. There I discovered my patients and how their lives and illnesses were intertwined. It is where I learned to be a doctor over the next three years. Mostly taught by my patients. When I told people that I worked at Cook County Hospital, their imaginations took off. They conjured up images of the Emergency Room; urban violence; the Saturday night "knife and gun club;" grit and despair; track-marked heroin addicts who shivered and vomited in withdrawal; toothless Skid Row winos who slept off weekend benders. Urban trauma, alcoholism and heroin punctuated the story of Cook County Hospital, but there was much more to the place.

Fantus Clinic was a Soviet-style yellow-brick and cement ambulatory office building appended to the west side of the main hospital by a corridor. Grey city pigeons lined up side by side on the concrete ledges outside the Fantus casement windows that faced Harrison Street as if mimicking the long lines of people inside the building. Across the street was a hamburger joint and Login's Medical Bookstore, where generations of doctors and students bought stethoscopes and medical textbooks. George, a grizzled, homeless schizophrenic, dressed Eskimo-like in layers of clothes and winter coats (even in summer), staked his claim to the Fantus Harrison Street entrance sometime in the late 1970s. All day he stood outside. At night he slept in the hospital. A de-facto doorman, he muttered and gesticulated at his internal tormentors. There was always a gaggle of assorted city people congregated near him puffing cigarettes under clouds of blue smoke. The Harrison Street bus rumbled to a stop in front of the Fantus entrance in twenty-minute cycles and let out load after load of passengers, a tide of humanity who surged past George into the Fantus lobby.

The lobby was clogged with patients. Standing. Limping. Shuffling. Sitting. On crutches. Rolling in wooden wheelchairs. Old. Young. Frail. Pregnant. In every nook and corner, they sprawled on benches. Jammed the elevators. They came to County to get outpatient care denied or unavailable elsewhere. Four hundred thousand each year. This was the County that did not make the evening news or the TV shows. Regular people who just needed to see a doctor and had nowhere else to go. They waited hours, endured rude clerks and inexperienced doctors like me. Lines ringed the clinic. They snaked down the hallways and around the corners. Lines for registration, for appointments, and even longer lines for the pharmacy. The patients armed themselves with bags filled with food. They were here for the long haul. Everyone knew you had to wait at County.

Most clinics had no set appointment times. The morning patients were told to come at 8:00 a.m. and the afternoon patients at 1:00 p.m. Once they showed up, it was first come first served. The oral surgery clinic had a perverse policy. They would treat only fifty patients daily. No appointments. Fantus' doors opened at 7:00 a.m. Patients with toothaches, loose teeth, oral tumors and mouth abscesses lined up in painful silence during the dark hours of the early morning. When the doors to Fantus were opened, it was like the starting gate at Arlington race track. They're off! The crowd scrambled through the open Fantus gates. Patients, some in wheelchairs, others with canes and crutches, raced to get to the Oral Surgery clinic to win one of the fifty prized slots that guaranteed a dentist would see them. This system had persisted through the years despite its inhumanity. Those who were too slow, too feeble, or too late to get one of those numbers would often leave, resigned to suffer and try again another day.

Why did County patients tolerate these waits and abusive conditions? Our patients declared that they came because County had "the best doctors." This was not true. There is no way we were the best. We were young, uninitiated, and worse, unsupervised. But many of our patients had been turned away from other institutions or had family or friends with the same experience. Maybe it was cognitive dissonance. Were their tributes to our medical prowess born of our lifesaving deeds or had they been conjured out of the cold fact that we were among the only doctors in the city who would see them without judgment? That it was worth the wait because County doctors were the best? Or maybe it was the only way they could justify to themselves the humiliation and abuse they endured. I felt unprepared to live up to my patients' expectations of me.

My first patient experience in clinic was inauspicious. There was no chart. Just a blank piece of yellow-lined paper. I called the patient into my cubicle and he sat in the chair, arms crossed, face gripped in an angry frown. A skinny, thin-haired middle-aged white guy, with bugged eyes. "I just need my phenobarbital, nothing more," he said. Epilepsy medication. He had been waiting for hours. The outpatients at Fantus had to change doctors every three years as a new batch of residents matriculated and the graduating ones departed. The luck of the draw. He scowled at me as if I was the short straw.

Maybe we would not have had the altercation had the chart been there. But it was missing. More often than not the patient charts never appeared. Maybe if the medication he was demanding had not been phenobarbital, a barbiturate and a controlled substance, I would not have challenged him. But with no chart, and no playbook, I was flustered. I felt the tension escalate in the tiny space as the blood rose to my face. He just wanted his scrip and nothing more. This was my first outpatient experience. I had never written a prescription before and this guy wanted me to take him at his word. For a barbiturate. "Now wait one minute, mister. Not so fast," I thought. I questioned him to be sure that he truly had the disease he claimed. "How do I know you have epilepsy?" I asked.

Purple splotches appeared on his neck and cheeks and rose to his ears with the challenge. His pupils narrowed. I had done it now. He stood up, now fully red-faced, fists clenched and yelled. His voice rebounded across the clinic. "Why would I make up epilepsy?" he screamed. "Give me my phenobarbital." I let loose in return. I might be young and inexperienced but I was not a pushover. I was nose to nose with my first patient—not what I had imagined when I opted for a career in primary care.

My mind raced as I considered my options. Phenobarbital was a controlled substance. What if he was a drug user? I gazed at the pile of charts in front of me. It was hot. The air was muggy. I had patients waiting for me in the hospital when I was done with clinic. Why would anyone fake epilepsy? He had a point. I had no frame of reference. I could not afford to get bogged down. I took a deep breath. "What the fuck?" I mused. I took his word, wrote out a prescription for three months of a medication I had only read about in a pharmacology book. He grabbed the scrip out of my hand as soon as I wrote it, eyebrows furrowed.

I was at a crossroads. Ready or not, here I was, "Presenting Dr. Ansell." A "real" doctor. And while I felt like a poseur, a fraud, I decided that despite my insecurity and inexperience, I needed to act as if I knew what the hell I was doing.

One month into my internship, on the West Side of Chicago, in a steamy corner of the fourth floor of Fantus Clinic, at the County Hospital. An epiphany. I suppressed a wave of panic and shoved my doubts aside. Oh. I got it. I was a "real" doctor now. The patients expected no less.

Somehow, that experience freed me up to dive in to outpatient medicine. My patients' lives were a window into a slice of American life I had never known—sharecroppers, wooden shacks on dusty backroads, back-breaking cotton picking for pennies a pound. Towns whose names littered civil rights history—Philadelphia, McComb, Indianola, Yahoo City, Little Rock, Montgomery, Birmingham. Life under Jim Crow. "Yes, suh. No, suh." The humiliation of survival in places where being black meant no chance for justice. The Illinois Central ride to Chicago. The promise of jobs. The disappointment of segregation and the urban violence that greeted them.

I learned about the lives of my patients in Chicago every week in that clinic. Hyper-segregated neighborhoods. Unsafe streets. Unemployment or backbreaking jobs in factories and foundries. Women followed when they walked around Loop clothing stores. My black male patients had all been stopped by the police for traffic violations—"Driving while black." They taught me the routine. Something I had never experienced myself. Flashing red lights. A floodlight blasts through the back window illuminating the interior of the car. Every black parent taught his or her children how to respond to a police stop. White kids were taught to trust the police. Black kids were taught to be cautious around the police. There was a routine that black men had learned to follow when stopped by the police. Open the window. Put your hands up. Easy does it. On top of the steering wheel where they could be seen as the cop approached the car. Sit still. The police flashlight aimed at the driver's side and then throughout the interior of the car. Look straight ahead. Don't move your hands unless the cop orders you to. No quick moves. Say "Yes, sir and no, sir." Do not argue.

This was just part of the reality of black life in Chicago. The hand of institutional racism was invisible to most white people, including my friends, who tended to avoid institutions or neighborhoods that catered to black people out of fear for their own safety or discomfort. My weekly session with my patients in the General Medicine Clinic heightened my sensitivity to the issues of race in America. In 1906, W.E.B. DuBois said, "The problem of the twentieth century is the problem of the color line." I was a middle-class white man from a small city in upstate New York. I had never been in a position to understand the meaning of these words until I was immersed in the lives of my patients that revealed their truth so powerfully and so tragically.

It did not take long for me to peel back the doctor-patient relationship more and discover other difficulties my patients faced. One of my patients was an elderly black woman, stoic and quiet, her hardscrabble life etched into the deep creases that traversed her face in such a way that her skin, had it been cloth, would have taken days to iron out. She sat quietly, in a button-down cotton dress, threadbare and almost colorless from many washings. Under it, her breasts sagged. Her steel wool wiry hair was iron gray and held in place with a bandana. She arrived in my office for a routine visit. Her blood pressure was through the roof. I leafed through the chart and noted it had been controlled in the past. I began to dig to see if I could identify a cause.

"How do you feel?" I probed.

"All right," she mumbled with her Arkansas accent.

"Are you having any chest pain or problems breathing?"

"No suh."

I tried another line of questioning before moving on. "Have you had any recent stress in your life?"

Jackpot. Her eyes welled. Her voice remained emotionless.

"My gran-chillin, got kilt. On my fron poich," she said.

Two teenage boys. Out of school. On their way to see her. Chased by gang members. They sprinted to her house. Bounded up the porch stairs. Frantic, the gang close behind, guns ablaze. Bullets ricocheted. Knock, knock, knock, they banged on the door. "Mama, mama, mama," they called for their grandma. She heard the shots and the banging, and thought the gang was trying to break in. She cowered in panic on the other side of the door, inches from her grandchildren.

"Ah was a-scared to open it. Ah din know it was them. Ah din know it was them," she repeated.

When she opened the door after the shooting stopped, she discovered the two young boys. Dead. Full of bullets, their blood joined in a pool on the porch. She wailed. "Jesus, Jesus, Jesus." Her blood pressure shot up. And remained high two weeks later.

If I had not asked, she would not have told me. I might have just adjusted her medicine and had her return in three months. I did not learn how to treat this in medical school. There was no medicine for grief, for the inevitability of urban violence. I felt powerless. I mumbled my sympathy and asked her to return in a month to recheck her blood pressure.

I heard similar stories from my other patients. The violent deaths of family members and friends, drugs and imprisonment. Children in gangs. Just about every man had a scar from a knife or bullet wound. Almost every woman had lost a close family member to violence. The names of lost loves and relatives were tattooed onto the arms and in the memories of my patients. Many years later, one of my patients lost her high-school-aged son in a drive-by shooting, a block away from home. It happened on a summer night in Chicago when thirty-one children were shot and eight died. He was killed when he pushed a girl out of the way of the bullets. My patient, the mother of the dead boy, climbed into bed with her mother, also my patient, and they held each other and cried together. Her two surviving children struggled at school. She developed diabetes and hypertension and some heart abnormalities. The grandmother's health deteriorated as well. How can these experiences not affect health and accelerate death in our patients? Each story left me, mouth agape, in shock and dismay. My condolences rang hollow.

Many years later, colleagues of mine conducted door-to-door health surveys in Chicago's poorest neighborhoods. More than a third of those surveyed had higher rates of depression, asthma, hypertension and smoking than those in white communities. Racism, poverty and violence took their toll. As an observer to the lives of my patients I could attest to the fact that poverty was as exhausting as it was deadly. I saw the damage it caused in the faces and bodies of my patients. These were painful lessons for me to learn as a twenty-six year old. But I could not imagine being anywhere else.

Sometimes, I got too close to my patients. Mary S. had severe rheumatoid arthritis and lung disease. She had spent her life cleaning white people's houses and raising their children. She moved to Chicago from Mississippi in the 1940s to find work. Now in her sixties, she had to quit work because of her advancing lung disease. She dragged a canister of oxygen with her to my office. In between gasps, she told me she wanted to get better and help raise my newborn son. She expressed no bitterness about her illness or about my inability to cure her. During her last hospitalization, she made one request. She lay in the hospital bed, her chest heaving to get air. We held hands.

"Doctor Ansen?" Her eyes sparkled. "Ah want ta see yo chile. Please, can ah see yo chile?" We hatched a plan. On the next Saturday morning, I brought my son to County Hospital for her to see. She came to the sixth floor window of the Medical A Building. I stood outside and held my infant son up over my head like a gift offering to the gods. She smiled and waved at us from the sixth floor window, oxygen tubes dangling from her nose. We waved back. I cried when she died a few days later.

I learned a lot from the patients. I was discovering the tools of medicine from them. Many of my patients and I grew up together. They had seen me become a father for the first time, and they consoled me when my father died. I had seen their children grow up, having children themselves. I had helped them through family crises, tragedies, diseases, and deaths. I had no idea in those first weeks and months of General Medicine Clinic how much I would grow from these relationships. I am on a first-name basis with many of my original patients. From them I gained insight into illness and the dignity with which people can face hardship that has helped me through difficult times in my life. I have taken care of three generations of some families, and have seen the destruction that poverty, poor diet, obesity, diabetes, and hypertension can unleash on a family's tree. I learned that sometimes giving hope or an embrace is as therapeutic as a drug. I sometimes measure my life progress by thinking of the people who have had an impact on my growth as a human being. My parents, my wife, my children, my friends and colleagues. I number my patients among them.

CHAPTER 8

ER

THE COUNTY EMERGENCY ROOM was a warren of examination areas and hallways located on the first floor of the main hospital. It was the O'Hare of emergency rooms, the busiest in the country. Maybe the world. While the General Medicine Clinic was a gentle immersion experience into the intricacies of outpatient medicine, the Emergency Room rotation at Cook County was the intern equivalent of being thrown to the sharks. My first day, I carried a small, black loose-leaf notebook in which I had written the treatments for common medical emergencies. Just in case.

On my first shift in the Emergency Room I headed toward the waiting room entrance off the main lobby of the hospital. A mistake. I should have taken the back way. The waiting room was packed. Standing room only. Some folks had waited for over a day to be seen. People were in the ER for many reasons. There were patients with true medical and surgical emergencies, who once seen were likely to be admitted to the hospital. Others were the walking wounded in need of diagnosis and treatment for conditions best taken care of in a doctor's office. Except there were no doctor's offices to see them. They came here instead. Others had been sent with prescriptions from doctors across the Chicago area for referral for specialty care or tests that could not be obtained elsewhere. Because you could not call Fantus Clinic and make an appointment for a doctor, the only way for a patient to see a specialist was to come to the ER, clutching these slips of paper in their hands. They did not know that after a day of waiting they would be referred to the purgatory of Fantus Clinic and have to endure months of further delays before they saw a specialist. It was a form of torture most of us would never tolerate. But if you were uninsured in Chicago, your options were limited. Some of the seats were occupied with the homeless and mentally ill who registered every day to guarantee themselves a seat to sleep, away from the harsh reality of Chicago's streets. Registration bought them protection from the County cops for twelve hours or more, the average wait time.

Patients strained to hear their names called by the nursing and clerical staff, some of whom had adopted hard-core surliness as protective armor against the constant inquiries. Some patients could not tolerate the wait. They collapsed and were rushed to the back. A quick trip to the head of the line. Sometimes the waiting room boiled over in mass anger and frustration. Especially when a doctor walked through.

As I sauntered in the first day, the tension in the waiting room was palpable. Voices rang out as patients saw an opportunity to plead their cases with me. They waved sheets of paper like pork belly traders at the Board of Trade. Asked me to get them seen. I stopped and listened but there was nothing I could do. I shook myself free. It was difficult to leave them empty-handed. From then on I avoided the ER waiting room when I could.

I straight-armed the double doors with the "No Admittance" sign that separated the waiting room from the work area. The ER was a long hallway with treatment rooms off the sides along its full length. Patients on gurneys were lined up, waiting to be seen. They clogged the hallway, some lay still under sheets while others moaned and writhed in pain. The first two doors on the right were examination rooms reserved for walk-in emergency patients. On the left was Room 101, known as the "Asthma Room." A little further down on the right was the Center—a bay that held four patients on stretchers. It's where the sickest patients were brought.

As interns, we had three responsibilities: to treat asthmatic patients in the Asthma Room, to see the less extreme walk-in emergencies or to perform surgical procedures in a room off the main ER known as the surgical dispensary. The orientation was brief. I was assigned to the Asthma Room. It was just me, my little black book and a nurse. The room had hospital beds and chairs for about fifteen patients. On a bad day all the beds were filled. Asthma is an inflammatory lung disease caused when the airways constrict and swell in response to an allergy, a virus or air pollution. It often begins suddenly and, if not treated, the patient can die. I had seen some asthma in medical school, but never a whole roomful of it.

The patient was wheeled in wheezing. Sweat trickled down his forehead and face as he strained to breathe. His pupils were dilated and the muscles of his neck retracted with every gasp. While the nurse obtained the vital signs, I listened to his lungs. The wheezing was audible even without a stethoscope. I ordered shots of epinephrine, a drug that we used to relax the airways. He received intravenous fluids, inhalation treatments, steroids and oxygen in short order as the nurse and I worked to calm his breathing down. The patient could go one of two ways. He would either respond to the medication and be able to go home in the next twelve hours or he would require hospitalization and days of treatment. Sometimes a patient's lungs were squeezed so tight by asthma that he would die if we did not act quickly. These patients sometimes required immediate mechanical ventilation and intensive care. Minutes could make a difference. There were no attending physicians to guide or supervise and the senior resident often had her hands full on the other side of the ER. But I learned from experience. We all did. I never treated so much asthma as I did that first year of residency in the ER. Dr. Kevin Weiss, a County resident who was a couple of years behind me in training, became a national expert on asthma, his interest likely piqued by his experience in Room 101. He studied asthma mortality and discovered that Chicago had the highest asthma death rate in the U.S. and that the deaths disproportionately targeted blacks and other minorities.

The surgical dispensary provided a similar immersion experience. The patients grasped numbered tags as they sat on hard benches and waited their turns. Rosie was the name of the nurse who ran the dispensary. Short, round and stuffed into her taut starched white nurse's uniform, she wore a County School of Nursing cap atop her thinning orange-dyed hair. She might have been the last nurse I met who still wore a nursing cap. A forty-year veteran of County, she was almost completely deaf when I met her and oblivious to the racket in the waiting area of the dispensary. A perfect match. She guided generations of interns through the rules of the dispensary. One of the last of the old-time County nurses, she told me that as a young nurse she had worked with Dr. Bernard Fantus, the County doctor whose name graced Fantus Clinic and who, in 1937, started the first blood bank in the world at County Hospital.

Rosie led me, like a sheep to slaughter, through the stuffed waiting room to the small procedure room off the waiting area, and behind a curtain. A row of dog-eared medical reference books were lined up on the stainless steel counter. I waited for Rosie to bring me a patient while she managed crowd control outside.

Pus bulged under the toenail of the first patient she brought in. It had to be removed. I had never done this before. I excused myself and scrambled to the main part of the ER to find the senior resident. He was bombarded by patients, harried and harassed. When I snagged his attention, he described how to anesthetize a toe or finger with local anesthetic by demonstrating on my hand. Lesson over. He was off to his next crisis. I sprinted back to the dispensary and opened one of the reference books. I found a section that described how to remove a toenail. I placed the book on the counter beside me. The corners of the pages were oily with finger marks of generations of interns like me who may have faced a similar predicament. I drew the anesthetic into the syringe and looked down at the picture in the book. "Close your eyes," I instructed the patient. "I am going to numb up your toe." This was more for my sake than his. I did not have the guts to tell him that I had never done this before. And I did not want him to see me reading from the book. My eyes darted between the diagram and his toe as I inserted the needle in the web between his toes and pushed in the contents of the syringe. Step by step, I followed the instructions in the book until I had the toenail off and the pus drained. The patient thanked me and hobbled out. I slouched back against the counter, relieved. You would have thought I had performed open heart surgery. "Next," Rosie yelled, as she poked her head through the curtain, and escorted another patient in.

"Hi, I am Dr. Ansell, how can I help you?"

The surgical dispensary learning process was trial by fire. An endless stream of patients. Lacerations. Abscesses. Foreign bodies. Nail removals. Bread and butter sort of stuff. I learned with a book on my lap; Rosie holding my hand. This was the medical equivalent of "paint by numbers." There was no formal teaching. It was not "see one, do one, teach one," the usual County training method, but rather "read one, do one, and pray." Not great for the patients. But over time, I gained confidence. I had other first experiences that month that tested my mettle. My first DOA. All of us experienced this first during our internships. And remembered it years later.

The loudspeaker blared the announcement:

"DOA at the back door; DOA at the back door."

The senior resident tracked me down and sent me to the ambulance entrance also known as the "back door" to assess the DOA. "What's a DOA?" I asked. "Dead on Arrival," he replied with a jaundiced sideways glance at me. One of the problems about being an intern was there was so much you did not know. After a while I learned that sometimes I just had to "do it." This was one of those times. "You have to go to the back door and pronounce a patient." Standard operating procedure. It was the intern's job in the Emergency Room. Part of the residency pecking order. I gulped, threw my stethoscope around my neck, and trembled my way to the back door by the ambulance dock. I had never "pronounced" a patient before. It is one thing to pry off a toenail after reading about it in a book; it is another to dispatch someone to the County morgue. I was too self-conscious to ask for help.

"A patient is not dead unless he is warm and dead." I remembered this from a medical school lecture. Patients whose bodies have been exposed to cold have to be warmed up before they can be pronounced dead. Hmm. Did I need to bring the body into the emergency room? What about resuscitation? Should I start CPR? Other than attending cardiac arrests in the hospital as part of a team, I had only one prior experience with death. Ten years earlier, in 1968. I was sixteen years old. An orderly. Pushing a supply cart through Our Lady of Lourdes Hospital for minimum wage, back in my hometown. An elderly lady died and the head nun asked me to deliver her corpse to the morgue. A first. I went to her room. She was covered with a sheet. The nurse and I lifted the body and placed it on the gurney. A tag with her name and date of birth hung from a blue big toe that stuck out from under the shroud. The elevator hummed as it descended to the basement. Just me and the cadaver. On an adolescent lark I decided to pretend to "pronounce" the patient in the elevator. I yanked back the sheet. The old woman was staring straight back at me through glassy eyes with an open toothless mouth. I yelped in fright and threw the sheet back over her head, my heart pounding in my throat. That was my first and last close encounter with death. Until County.

I trekked to the back of the Emergency Room where a brick covered structure connected the driveway outside to the emergency room. There was room for two ambulances and this is where the most seriously ill patients arrived at County. A door near the police station led out of the ER "back door" to the ambulance dock. I pulled the door and loped down the stairs to the tarmac. But there was no ambulance, just a police paddy wagon, engine running, the words "To Serve and Protect" emblazoned on the side. Two of "Chicago's finest" stood smoking cigarettes. Their open leather jackets barely covered guts that protruded over patent leather gun belts. The air was stale and smelled of cigarette smoke and exhaust.

"Hi. I'm Dr. Ansell, what's up?" I felt self-conscious and intimidated in their presence. My long curly hair and moustache blared "Hippie!" They appeared nonplussed and bored.

"Hey, Doc, we found dis John Doe. Down on Wahshintin Street. Skid Row. He's dead as a doornail," one of the cops said, as he sucked a long draw of his Marlboro and blew the smoke out through his mouth and nose. He pronounced Washington as "Wahshintin" in the Chicago vernacular that bobbles vowels and consonants like the Cubs' infield blows double plays. There were a handful of flop houses on Madison and Washington Streets where winos and addicts rented spaces. TB was rampant there, as were overdoses.

The other cop unlatched the back door to the paddy wagon to reveal a fiftyish white man on the steel bed of the truck, head facing out, eyes closed. He was grizzled, with an asphalt-colored beard and moustache. A dark knit cap covered his head like a helmet. Yellow teeth protruded through a partially opened mouth. Multiple layers of clothes gave him a robust and hardy look. He appeared asleep.

I felt awkward, in over my head. Did these cops know that I was an amateur? A warm rush of blood rose to my face as the two Chicago cops eyeballed me and awaited my next move. I bent over and stared face to face with John Doe. I put my ear to his mouth to see if I could hear him breathe. Nah. I listened for a heart beat. I fumbled with my stethoscope and bent over John Doe, unzipped his jacket and placed the stethoscope over his layers of clothes. How long should I listen? I did not know. Time passed in slow motion. The only sound I heard through the stethoscope was the beat of my own heart in my ears. "Oh shit," I thought. After what seemed to be a respectful amount of time, I furrowed my brow and put my best "serious doctor look" on my face. I turned to the cops, nodded and mumbled, *sotto voce*, "Yeah, he's dead." They had me sign a piece of paper to that effect. John Doe went to the County morgue. I tossed and turned that night, hoping I was right.

CHAPTER 9

I Call It Murder

SIX MONTHS INTO MY INTERNSHIP, things began to spiral out of control. We were beleaguered. Not just from the residency training, but also from the outside world. The governance of County Hospital was in disarray. The ten-year conflict between the County Board, which had fiscal control of the hospital, and the Governing Commission, the independent board that operated the hospital, heated up and came to a head. The County controlled the purse strings. The Governing Commission controlled the jobs. It was a squeeze play. The Democratic Machine controlled the County Board, which had the hospital and its legions of patronage jobs yanked from its control ten years earlier. And the County Board wanted them back. So they hatched a plan to bring the hospital to its knees by withholding funds. It was political corruption of the highest order.

The patients and staff were caught in the middle. Supplies were short; tests delayed; staff was on edge; workers laid off; tempers short. Yet the patients kept coming. The *Chicago Tribune* fueled the flames with editorials that called for the hospital to be shuttered. Our jobs and training were at risk as well as the lives of our patients. As the conflict escalated in late 1978, some of our fellow residents jumped ship and applied to train elsewhere for the following July. A showdown was inevitable.

The atmosphere was hot with political fervor and activity. Our meetings were raucous, heated and argumentative as we strategized about what to do. To paraphrase Abbie Hoffman's comment about the Chicago Seven trial ten years earlier: we could not agree on lunch, let alone strategy. There were people from every political persuasion from left to right. We all agreed that we had to keep the hospital open. Gordy Schiff and Mardge Cohen had joined with others to form the "Committee to Save Cook County Hospital." The group's purpose was to organize patients, doctors and staff to speak out at County Board meetings. Jim Schlosser, my friend from medical school, argued that saving Cook County was not enough, "We need to transform Cook County Hospital as well." Why would we want to save a place that was so broken, he argued. If we organized, it had to be to turn it into something better.

For the black physicians, led by Dr. Linda Rae Murray, the fight between the mostly black independent Governing Commission and the mostly white County Board was a replay of the old race politics of Chicago and a blatant power grab. Linda accepted the task as president of the House Staff union in July of 1979. I served on the House Staff executive committee and worked on the house staff newsletter. We had set up a silkscreen press in the house staff offices on the second floor of Karl Meyer Hall to print posters that we waved during the demonstrations downtown. "Keep County Open. Health Care for People, Not Profit," they said. I don't remember how often we demonstrated that year, but when we finished our morning rounds we would take the short El trip downtown, a sea of white coats, to hold brief, poster-waving protests at Daley Plaza across from the County Building. "Keep County open," we chanted at lunchtime and returned to the hospital to take care of our patients. We showed up in force at the public hearings down at the County Building.

Many of us viewed the troubles at County Hospital as just a manifestation of the broader unresolved conflicts in Chicago and the U.S. around race, health and poverty. Chicago was one of the most segregated cities in the U.S. It was not by chance that it was so racially divided, but by policy and perverse design. Martin Luther King had moved to the West Side of Chicago in 1966 to highlight the segrega-

tion of schools and housing in Chicago. Panic peddling by unscru-
pulous real estate agents led to widespread white flight shortly after
blacks began to move into these formerly all white neighborhoods.
Unable to obtain mortgages through local banks or the Federal
Housing Authority because of racist lending practices, black home
owners were forced to enter into prohibitive purchase contracts with
the same real estate agents who had bought the housing at rock-bot-
tom prices from fleeing whites. Many black homeowners were evicted
when they could not meet the terms of these crooked contracts and
the same real estate agents resold the reclaimed properties over and
over again, driving neighborhood instability and deterioration.
Businesses fled the neighborhoods as well. Many of the businesses that
remained were destroyed during the riots on the West Side of Chicago
after Martin Luther King's assassination in 1968. Landlords burned
down apartment buildings as well to collect insurance money, leaving Chicago's ghettos with more abandoned buildings and empty lots
than existed after the great Chicago fire of 1871.

The former Mayor, Richard J. Daley, who denied the presence of
ghettos in Chicago, had used federal highway and housing dollars to
separate the white southwest side of Chicago from the black south-
east side of the city. The eight-lane Dan Ryan Expressway was built
down the middle of Wentworth Avenue, the traditional battleground
between Daley's Irish Bridgeport neighborhood and the expanding
black neighborhood to the east. An eight-lane moat with train tracks
down the middle, it created a physical barrier between white and
black Chicago. On the black side of the Dan Ryan, the Robert Taylor
Homes, the largest segregated high-rise housing project in the world,
also built with federal housing dollars, condemned two generations of
blacks to lives of hyper-segregated poverty and violence.

The police in Chicago were also known for their brutal methods.
In 1968, the whole world watched as the Chicago police attacked
crowds of young anti-war demonstrators during the Democratic
National Convention in what was later called a "police riot" by an
independent commission. No one was watching in 1969 when Fred

Hampton, a Black Panther leader in Chicago, was murdered in his bed eight blocks from County Hospital at 4:00 a.m. during a police raid ordered by Illinois State's Attorney Edward Hanrahan and the FBI. It would be several years later that we would learn about the torture of black suspects by a Chicago Police Commander during the 1970s and 1980s in a South Side police district. Commander John Burge and other officers in the Chicago Police Department systematically tortured prisoners with burns, electric shocks to the genitals, and other brutal methods to obtain false confessions for capital crimes. Despite overwhelming evidence of the torture, it took thirty years before Burge faced prosecution and then only in Federal Court. As the courts overturned a number of convictions of Death Row inmates whose confessions were coerced by torture, the death penalty was initially suspended in Illinois, then outlawed in March 2011.

We viewed the attacks on the hospital through the lens of Chicago's racial history. Because County Hospital served black people, Latinos and the uninsured, we believed that the hospital and its clinics would never receive enough resources or generate the outrage from the civic community to repair the conditions there. We were angry and determined to take matters into our own hands. The hospital was in decrepit shape. Quality of care was spotty. Over fifty years earlier, in 1927, the American College of Surgeons called for the hospital to be rebuilt. Now it slithered toward closure with no replacement in sight. Our anxiety was well-founded. In Philadelphia, Mayor Frank Rizzo had closed the famous public hospital, Philadelphia General, just two years before, and closures of other public hospitals around the country had become more common. We knew we faced a similar threat and were desperate to do anything to save and rebuild Cook County Hospital.

There was dysfunction everywhere we looked. The structural problems at the old hospital were life-threatening—no inside fire escapes, no sprinklers, electrical wiring problems. The administration knew about it. They were cited by the regulators but had never bothered to fix the wiring. There was no back-up generator in case of a power failure. Once, the unthinkable happened. The electrical power went out in the medical ICU. The room went black. Nothing worked. Nine out of the ten ventilators stopped. The patients were dependent on the machines to breathe. Doctors were called from around the hospital to help. Until the power was restored an hour later doctors and nurses stood in the dark and pumped air by hand into the patients' lungs. Two patients died after the black-out was over but the medical examiner reported that it was from natural causes.

While this was an extreme example of "County gone wild," every day the patients and staff suffered indignities because the hospital did not function normally. The disastrous medical conditions and supply shortages were not a new phenomenon at County Hospital; they had been the norm since its inception. It was how the poor had always been treated. A century before, during a period when the liquor bills for the hospital exceeded the medical supply costs, a patient died when a rotten piece of catgut supplied for a surgery snapped and leaked feces into the abdominal cavity of the patient. His surgeon, the famous Danish-born pathologist, Dr. Christian Fenger, performed the autopsy in the autopsy amphitheater surrounded by dozens of students and colleagues who peered down from their roosts above. The natural light from large windows illuminated the procedure. The patient's abdomen was splayed open and when Dr. Fenger discovered the piece of rotten catgut born of administrative malfeasance and corruption, he looked up from his dissection and shook his fist in the direction of the warden's office. "Reformers?" he shouted in frustration. "No, murderers!" So the dysfunction and frustration we were experiencing in the late 1970s was no different from that experienced by legions of doctors and nurses before us. But we decided to take action.

During the period from 1978 to 1979 some of our anger was directed toward Presbyterian-St. Luke's Hospital, the private hospital across the street from County. Presbyterian was a convenient foil. The juxtaposition of these two hospitals on Chicago's Harrison Street represented everything we thought was wrong with the two-tiered health-care system in the U.S. Presbyterian was a private academic medical center that served an insured and largely white population while, across the street and a world away, County served the downtrodden, the uninsured and a mostly black population. Presbyterian was planning a new hospital while we were fighting to keep our eighty-year-old building open. To add fuel to the fire, Presbyterian's CEO, Dr. James Campbell had authored a report, "The Campbell Plan," that envisioned the shuttering of County Hospital and the distribution of indigent care across the city hospitals. While an egalitarian notion, no one believed that anyone wanted "County" patients, least of all Presbyterian. The Metropolitan Chicago Health Care Council jumped on the bandwagon and also proposed razing County Hospital and shipping the indigent patients to other hospitals.

In the 1960s and 1970s, as the West Side of Chicago became the destination for increasing numbers of African Americans migrating from the South, private hospitals in Chicago developed strategies to seal themselves off from the "unfavorable" demographics of the changing West Side. At some Chicago hospitals, like Presbyterian, indigent black obstetric patients were kept on separate floors from insured patients, a practice that was ended when it was exposed by medical students. Many hospitals closed their public clinics to minimize their exposure to the uninsured. Because the uninsured were more likely to be black and Latino than white, these policy decisions took on racial overtones in Chicago, one of the most racially divided cities in America.

The first demonstration against Presbyterian occurred in 1978, soon after I arrived in Chicago. Presbyterian was dedicating a new cancer treatment center. A group of County house staff marched down Harrison Street, twenty to thirty strong, and stood across the street to protest. The point of this demonstration was to express anger that a new cancer center was being built at Presbyterian while our patients at County suffered the humiliation of outdated facilities and a potential shutdown. The folks at "Pres" had no idea why County house staff were raining on their party. A couple of former "Rush-Pres" medical students, now County residents, tried to shout down the speeches but the police arrested them and threw them into a paddy wagon. Not a pretty scene. But it was a sign of the times that a group of County docs were willing to take to the streets at the drop of a hat.

As the crisis at County heightened to a fever pitch, Presbyterian inadvertently precipitated another demonstration when it closed down a short strip of Paulina Street. The winter of 1978–79 had blanketed the region with blizzard conditions and ground the city to a halt. I was stuck at the hospital for three consecutive days as public transportation and auto traffic were shut down. The "Machine" candidate for mayor, Michael Bilandic, was being challenged by upstart Jane Byrne, and she was able to make the city's inaction during the blizzards a campaign issue. She was looking for ways to publicize her campaign. Presbyterian's precipitous closure of Paulina Street provided an opportunity for her to appear anti-establishment.

During the spring of 1979, with no opportunity for public comment, Presbyterian had persuaded the Chicago City Council to sell them a small stretch of Paulina Street adjacent to the site where a new wing of Presbyterian Hospital was being erected. Immediately, Presbyterian barricaded the street. However, Paulina Street was also the main ambulance route to the County Hospital Emergency Room from the West Side. Now the ambulances were diverted to a longer route. One patient died en route as reported by the *Chicago Sun Times* columnist, Mike Royko. True or not, we were in an uproar at County, and so the House Staff Association along with the Nurse's Union planned a demonstration to protest this street closure. The CEO of Presbyterian was hung in effigy over the barricaded street. Leaflets, posters and buttons were designed with the slogan, "Open Paulina, Close Pres." Jane Byrne, just weeks before the Chicago mayoral election, promised to re-open the street if elected. "Open Paulina!" one group of marchers chanted. "Close Pres!" another group replied, as hundreds of white-coated doctors and nurses marched down Harrison Street chanting and waving signs At the front of the protest marched the next Mayor of Chicago, Jane Byrne. Byrne was elected Mayor and when the new Presbyterian wing opened, Jane Byrne was there on the podium to dedicate it. Paulina remained closed.

The final demonstration was as spontaneous as it was bold. One sunny October day in 1979, a parade of patients in wooden wheelchairs were rolled out of the County Emergency Room and pushed down Harrison Street towards "Pres." Anxiety at County Hospital was high. There were more layoffs. The Governing Commission asked the County Board for more funding. The Board refused to give another cent until they wrested back control of the hospital from the independent commission. For three consecutive pay periods we were told we might not get paid. They had run out of money. At the last minute they were able to make payroll, but still we lurched towards the precipice. It was so unnecessary. The Republican Governor of Illinois and the Democratic President of the Cook County Board were using the funding crisis to eliminate the independent Governing Commission. Three hundred of us had rallied at the Daley Center the previous Saturday chanting, "Save County Hospital!" But no amount of protesting could prevent the inevitable from occurring.

Then we hit rock bottom. On payday, Wednesday, October 16, 1979, the Governing Commission could not make payroll. No one at the hospital received a paycheck. The tension was at a fever pitch. I was on the "diarrhea" ward in the Children's Hospital treating a floor full of sick babies when I heard the news about the payless payday. The hospital leadership asked the workers to stay on the job. It was not an option to abandon our patients. As word of the crisis spread across the hospital, a rally was quickly called for noon. It was a sunny fall afternoon, one of those cloudless Chicago autumn days with azure blue skies and warm breezes. Dr. Linda Rae Murray, the House Staff President announced that we were going to close down the clinics and the Emergency Room but continue to take care of inpatients. Someone from the crowd proposed that we remove patients from the County Emergency Room and escort them to Presbyterian Hospital across the street. "Let's see if the private hospitals will treat our patients," we said. Dozens of sign-waving County House Staff and other employees descended on the ER and told bewildered patients that they were being taken to Presbyterian. Some were pushed in rickety, wooden wheelchairs. Others walked over, escorted by white-coated young doctors.

The crowd numbered well over 200 including the baffled patients. Television crews and the print media were on hand. After over a hundred people entered Presbyterian, security guards barred the doors. Presbyterian to its credit agreed to treat all the patients, but six patients came back to County when they were not assured that the care would be free. Some house staff at Presbyterian were furious with the County doctors for using the patients to make a political point. It was a desperate tactic, and wrong to involve the patients. But it was a manifestation of how hopeless we felt.

Downtown, the next week, a group of activists from County marched around the Cook County Building chanting and waving posters. Inside, fifteen doctors and community activists held a sit-in at the Cook County Board President's office and were arrested. Meanwhile, the chairman of Pediatrics at County took a more civilized approach and called around the city to find other hospitals to take in the sixty-five high-risk neonates in County's neonatal intensive care unit. He could only find placement for five. Eventually a back-room deal restored funding to the hospital. The County and the State found 4.8 million dollars that kept the hospital operating and the staff paid. The Governing Commission was thrown out, all its administrators fired and the County Board took over the operation of the hospital. Patronage politics was back in full force. Cook County Hospital had slipped to the edge of a chasm only to be thrust back into the jaws of the Democratic Machine.

During this same period, the BBC arrived from London to film a documentary about Cook County Hospital. They interviewed Dr. Linda Rae Murray. Linda, in addition to being the House Staff President, was the unofficial "dean" of the black physicians at County. Linda was more comfortable in the leadership of the Black Physicians Association but realized the importance of taking on the presidency of the union. Many of us felt that she could speak more directly to the concerns of black Chicagoans than a young white doctor with no connection to the community. Linda had no hesitation in taking it to County Board politicians. "Let me make one thing perfectly clear!" She would lecture the County Commissioners during budget hearings, as her finger jabbed the air for emphasis. The white commissioners viewed her as an angry black militant. The black commissioners did not want her rocking the boat.

In spite of her own militancy, Linda was cautious about some of the tactics of the "crazy white folks" as she referred to those of us who might stay at County for a few years, rile things up and then leave the hospital and the black communities of Chicago stuck in the mire of segregation and dysfunction. She had been a medical student at County during the House Staff strike four years earlier and active in political organizations for much of her adult life. She paid a price for speaking up that none of us faced. Her leadership role with the house staff union during this period so angered and frightened the downtown politicians that she was the only one of us who was denied an attending physician position after training. It would be many years before she would be allowed to return.

The BBC interview was classic. Linda was asked about the consequences of the hospital's conditions and funding deficiencies on the health of black people. She responded with a succinct, "I call it murder." "I Call it Murder" became the title of the BBC documentary that aired in England later that year. Many of us agreed with her diagnosis.

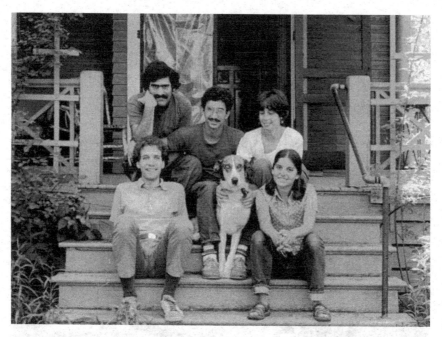

Our house in Syracuse, New York in 1977. Back row: left to right, Barry Abrams, the author, and Cate Stika. Front row: left to right, Stuart Kiken and the author's wife, Paula Grabler (who completed an internship at County in the 1990s). Cate was the only one who did not train at County. Three other Syracuse medical students (not pictured) also came to train at County. *(Courtesy Barry Abrams, MD)*

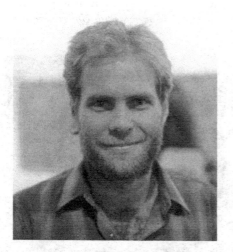

Jim Schlosser, another member of the "Syracuse Group," came with us to County in 1978. *(Courtesy Jim Schlosser, MD)*

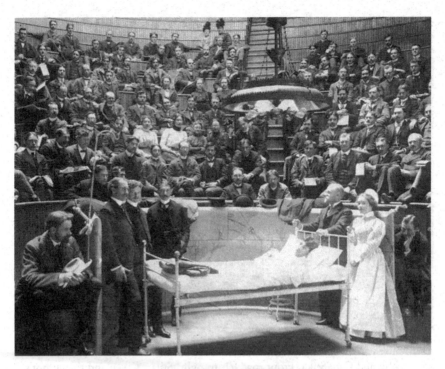

The old Cook County Hospital ampitheater circa late 1800s. Top: Dr. James Herrick, on the right with the beard, the first scientist to describe sickle cell anemia, identified the sickled cells in a blood smear taken from a Cook County medical student with the disease. Bottom: Cadavers being dissected by Dr. Christian Fenger (center) who once accused the management of Cook County Hospital of being "murderers." *(Courtesy Rush University Medical Center Archives)*

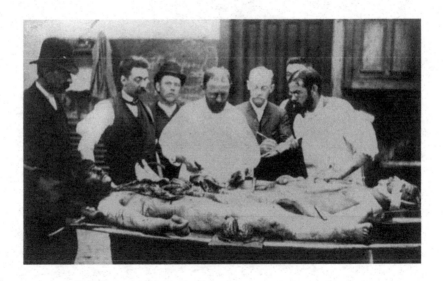

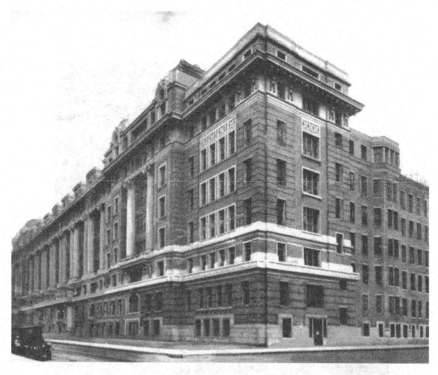

Cook County Hospital, 1914. *(Courtesy Cook County Health and Hospital System Archives)*

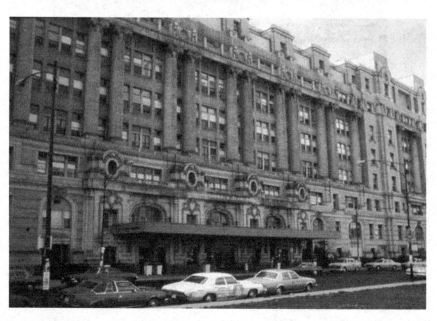

Cook County Hospital, sometime in the late 1970s or early 1980s. *(Courtesy Stuart Kiken, MD)*

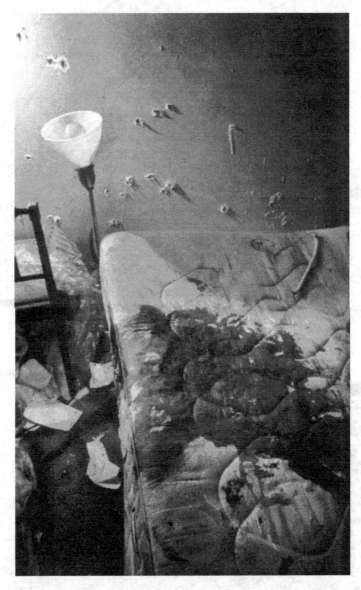

In 1969, Black Panther leader Fred Hampton was assassinated while sleeping in his apartment located near County Hospital, in what later was found to be a police and FBI conspiracy. The other victims of the attack were taken to Cook County Hospital for treatment of their wounds. *(Courtesy Paul Sequeira)*

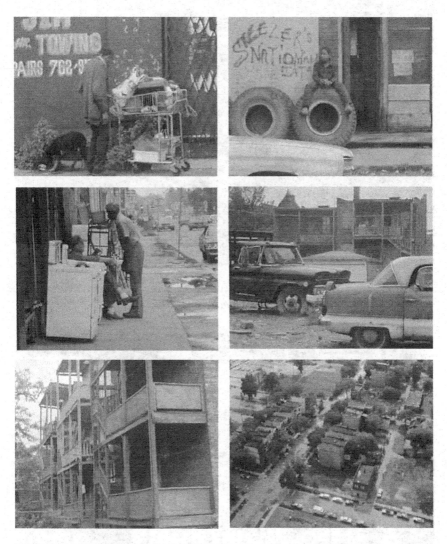

The neighborhoods around Cook County Hospital were run down, hyper-segregated, and over crowded with dilapidated housing stock. There were more empty lots in Chicago in 1978 than there were after the Great Chicago Fire of 1871. *(Courtesy author)*

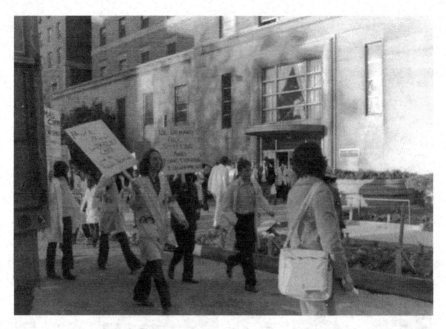

House staff strike in 1975, residents picketing outside of Cook County Hospital. *(Courtesy Cook County Health and Hospital System Archives)*

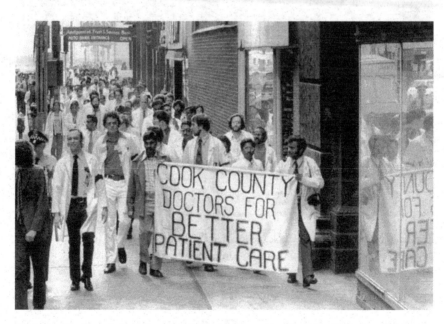

House staff officers on strike, marching downtown in the fall of 1975 in defiance of a back-to-work order. After the strike was over, seven young physicians were sentenced to Cook County Jail for contempt of court. *(Courtesy* Chicago Tribune*)*

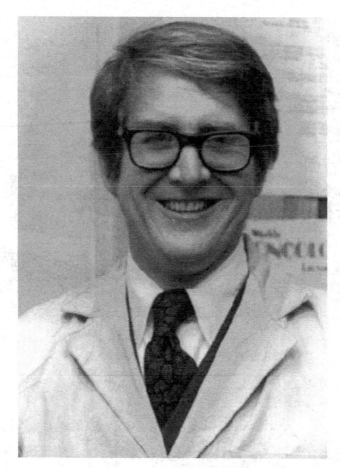

Dr. Quentin Young, Chair of the
Department of Medicine at Cook
County Hospital, was a role model for
us because of his involvement in the
civil rights and anti-war movements of
the 1960s. *(Courtesy Cook County Health
and Hospital System Archives)*

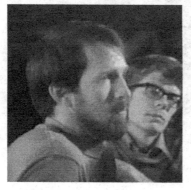

Dr. Jack Raba, president of the House
staff, foreground, at a press conference
before being jailed for ten days at Cook
County Jail for defying a court injunction
of the 1975 House staff strike. He later
became medical director of the health
services at the jail. *(Courtesy author)*

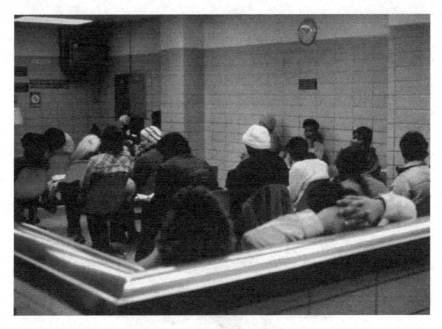

Crowded waiting room, Cook County Emergency Room. *(Courtesy Gordon Schiff, MD)*

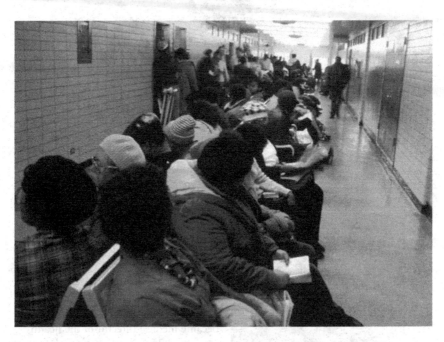

Fantus Clinic hallway, packed with patients. *(Courtesy Gordon Schiff, MD)*

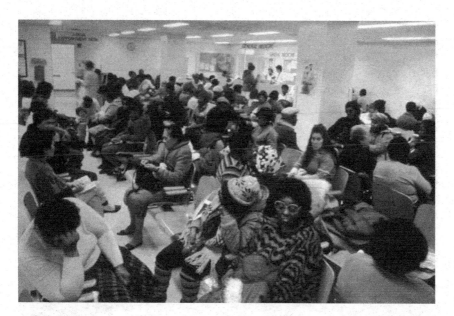

The General Medicine Clinic waiting room. Patients could wait hours before they were seen. Many brought food and were prepared to wait as long as it took to see the County doctors. *(Courtesy Gordon Schiff, MD)*

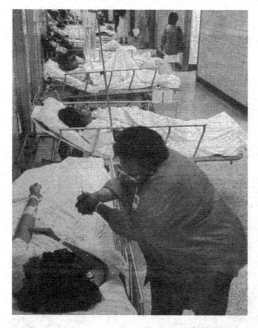

The emergency room hallway was usually lined up with patients. *(Courtesy author)*

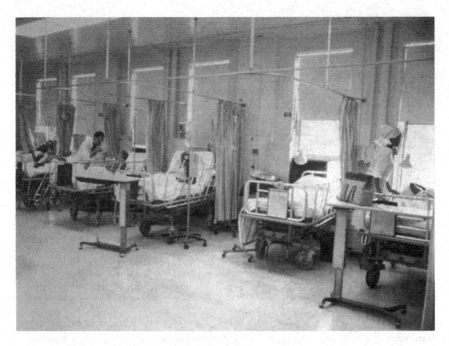

The open wards at Cook County. These were state of the art at the turn of the twentieth century but by the late 1970s were unusual in U.S. hospitals. *(Courtesy David Goldberg, MD)*

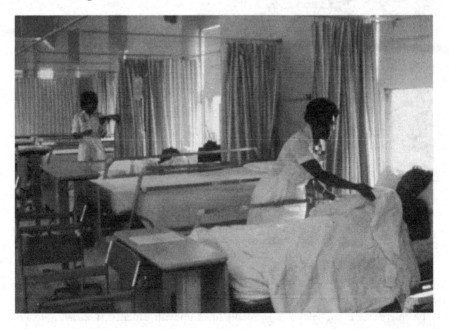

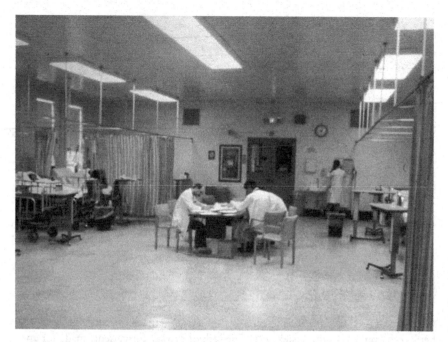

Top: Residents working at the table on Ward 35, the admitting ward at Cook County. This ward was the saving grace for medical residents because on admitting night and there was a feeling that we were all in it together. Bottom: (Left) Reba MacLin, the evening admitting clerk on Ward 35. She ruled the ward with a combination of "tough love" and warmth. (Right) A resident rounding on the OB ward, pushing a chart rack. *(Courtesy Stuart Kiken, MD)*

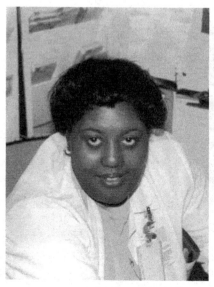

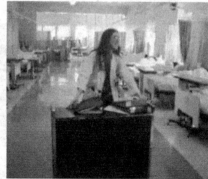

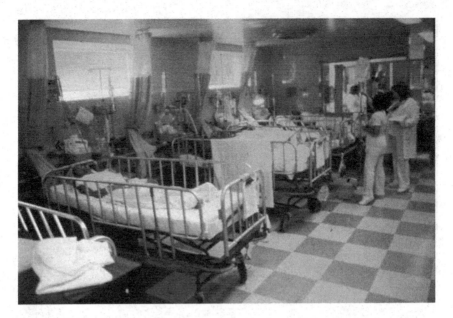

Open wards: because the nursing care was spotty, sometimes patients who were better off would help the sicker ones. The lack of privacy for patients made for an unpleasant recovery experience. *(Courtesy David Goldberg, MD)*

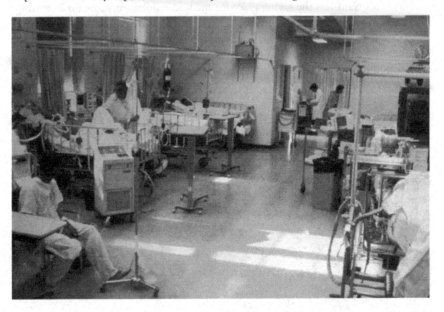

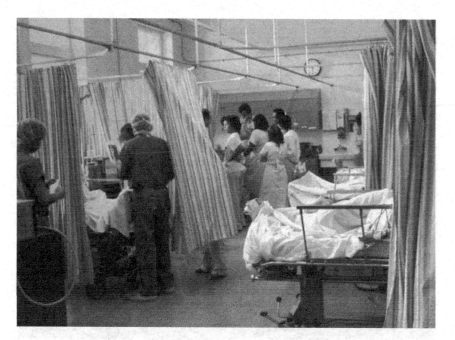

Top: Cook County Hospital Trauma Unit. Bottom: A group of nurses and doctors working feverishly on a sick patient in the Cook County Emergency Room. It was one of the busiest in the U.S. and the residents ran the show. In the late 1970s there were few attending physicians to provide oversight or guidance. *(Courtesy Cook County Health and Hospital System Archives)*

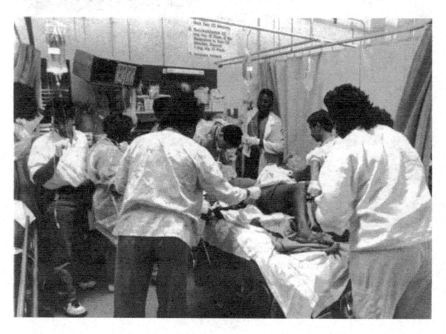

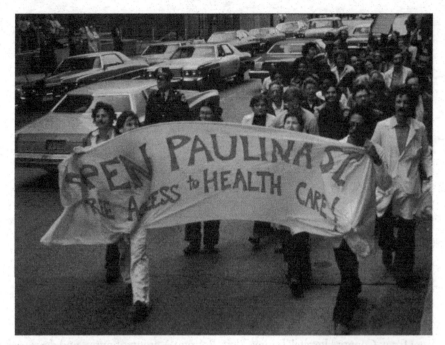

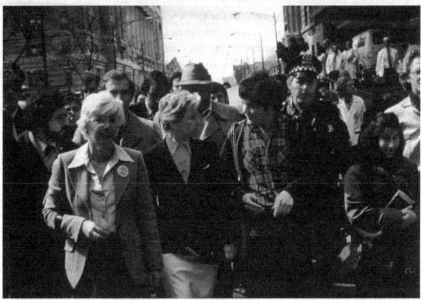

Top: Protesting the closing of Paulina Street, the main ambulance thoroughfare to the Cook County Hospital Emergency Room. Bottom: Upstart Chicago mayoral candidate, Jane Byrne, leads the march against the closing of Paulina Street, hoping the attention she gets will help her election. She pledged that if elected mayor she would re-open the street. *(Courtesy Babs Waldman, MD)*

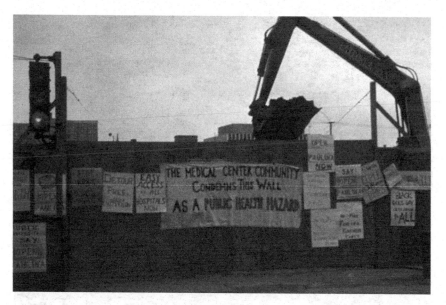

Top: The construction wall at Paulina Street with sign, "The Medical Center Community Condemns this Wall." Bottom: (Left) A protester with homemade sign. *(Courtesy Babs Waldman, MD)* (Right) Jane Byrne was elected mayor of Chicago, changed sides and one year later keynoted the dedication of a new hospital building at Rush-Presbyterian Hospital. Paulina Street remained closed. *(Courtesy Rush University Medical Center Archives)*

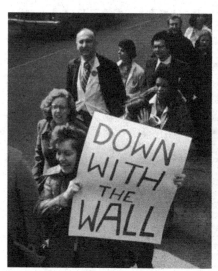

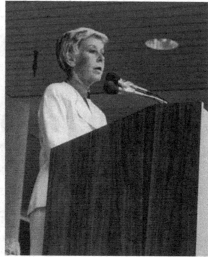

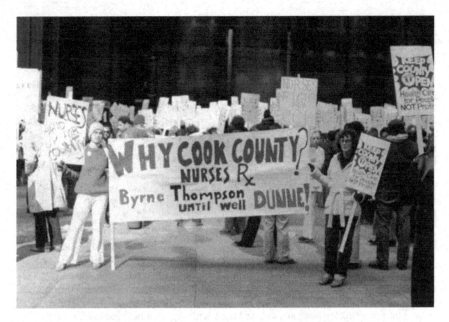

Rally in downtown Chicago in October 1979 calling on politicians to find the money to save the hospital. Hospital workers went the whole month not knowing if they would get paid. *(Courtesy Babs Waldman, MD)*

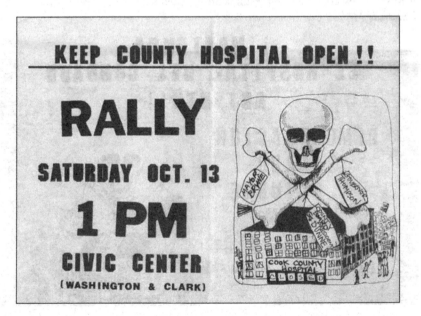

Poster calling Cook County Hospital workers to a rally to save the hospital. We were doctors by day and "moonlighted" as activists in the off hours. *(Courtesy author)*

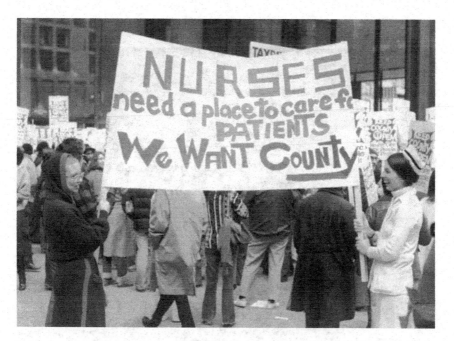

Top: Nurses demonstrating in downtown Chicago to keep County Hospital open. *(Courtesy Babs Waldman, MD)* Bottom: (Left) Dr. Linda Rae Murray, president of the House Staff Association, in 1979. During an interview with the BBC she was asked to describe what was happening to the patients at County. She replied, "I call it murder." *(Courtesy author)* (Right) The author as a young house staff physician. *(Courtesy Peter Orris, MD)*

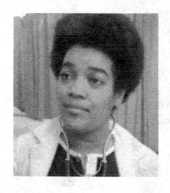

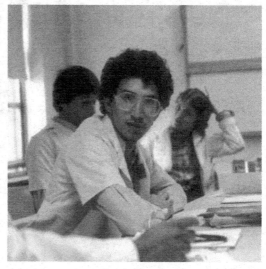

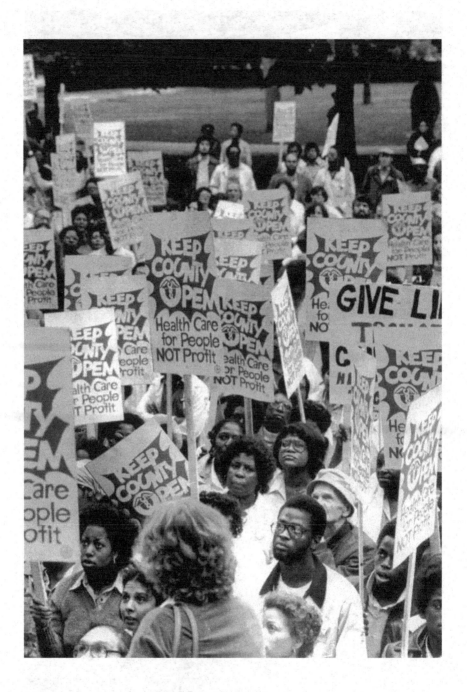

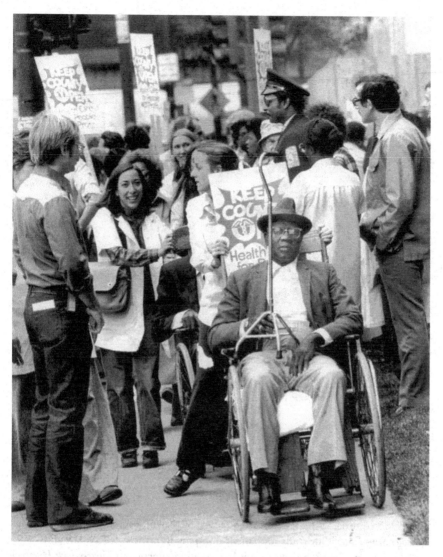

In October, 1979 the County Hospital could not make payroll. It was out of money. A spontaneous demonstration errupted, and a decision was made to close down County's Emergency Room and wheel patients over to Presbyterian Hospital. Opposite: Rally outside of County Hospital. Above: County doctors, including Mardge Cohen, MD (first woman on the left, pushing a patient in a wheelchair) take patients from County to Presbyterian. *(Courtesy* Chicago Tribune*)*

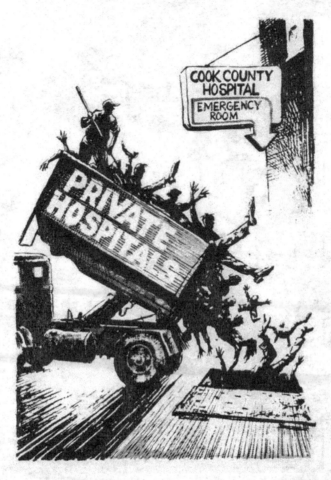

This 1985 editorial cartoon about the practice of patient dumping appeared in the *Chicago Sun-Times*. Our study on patient dumping influenced federal law and ended the most heinous aspects of this longstanding practice. *(Courtesy Jack Higgins)*

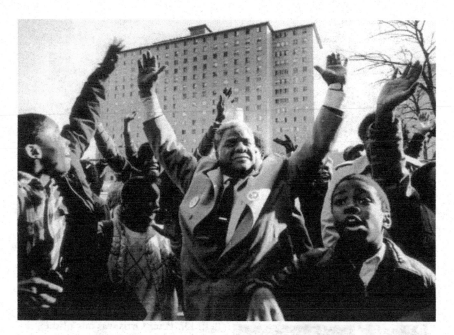

Harold Washington was elected as the first black Mayor of Chicago in 1983. His Democratic primary victory the day before a Cook County Board budget hearing was thought to have helped fund the Breast Cancer Screening Program at County Hospital. *(Courtesy* Chicago Tribune*)*

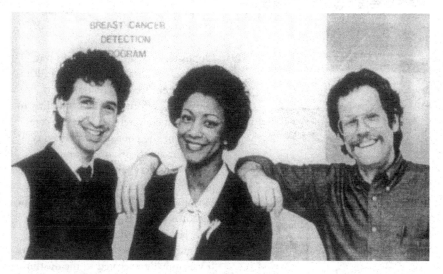

(Left to right) The author, Dr. Loretta Lacey and Dr. Steve Whitman worked on the Breast Cancer Screening Program at County. It was one of the first programs in the U.S. to focus on the alarming disparity in breast cancer mortality based on race. *(Courtesy author)*

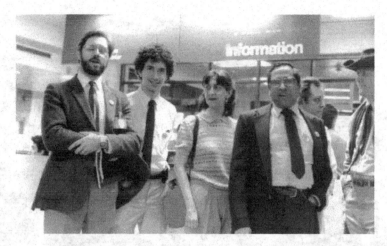

A group of attending physicians (including the author, second from left) on the day we turned in signed union cards for our first attempt to organize an attending union at Cook County Hospital in 1985. *(Courtesy Peter Orris, MD)*

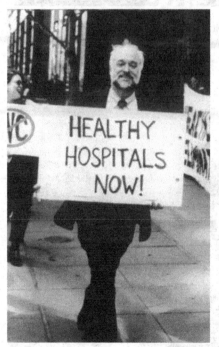

Left: Dr. Peter Orris was one of the leaders of the unionization attempts for attending physicians. It was not until 2008, twenty-three years after the first attempt to unionize, that the attending physicians at John H. Stroger, Jr. Hospital of Cook County were allowed to unionize. *(Courtesy Peter Orris, MD)*

Opposite: A coalition of unions published a "Proposal for a Public Health Care System for Cook County" in 1985. This effort was one of the first to envision a comprehensive health care system for the poor in Cook County. It called for a network of community health centers, a South Side public hospital and building a new Cook County Hospital on the West Side campus. The author is pictured on the front along with Jackie Dillard, one of the nurses who ran the Breast Screening Program. It was quickly relegated to the dustbin. It would be almost two more decades before a new Cook County Hospital would be built. *(Courtesy author)*

Proposal for a Public Health Care System for Cook County

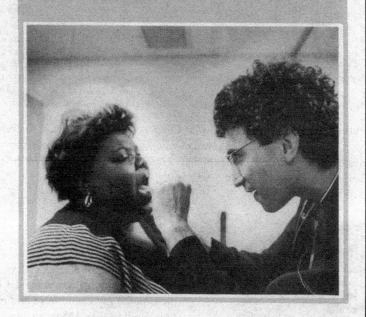

Cook County Hospital Union Coalition:

House Staff Association of Cook County Hospital
Illinois Nurses Association
Licensed Practical Nurses Association of Illinois
American Federation of State, County & Municipal Employees
Pharmacists Association/RWDSU
National Union of Hospital & Health Care Employees/1199

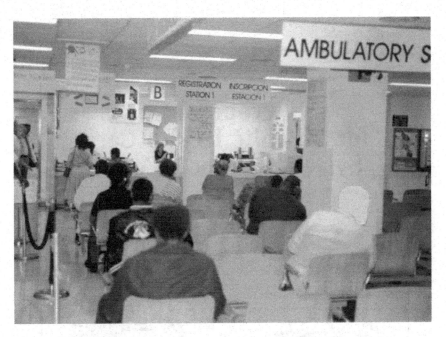

The waiting room at the walk-in clinic at County. This clinic represented every-thing that was wrong with the U.S. health care system. Most of the patients who used this clinic needed primary or specialty care that was not available in their neighborhoods. *(Courtesy Gordon Schiff, MD)*

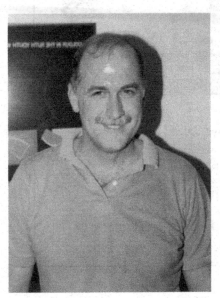

Ron Sable, a health activist, leader in the Chicago gay community, and two-time candidate for Alderman, was the co-founder of the HIV/AIDS clinic at County. He died of AIDS in 1993. *(Courtesy Stuart Kiken, MD)*

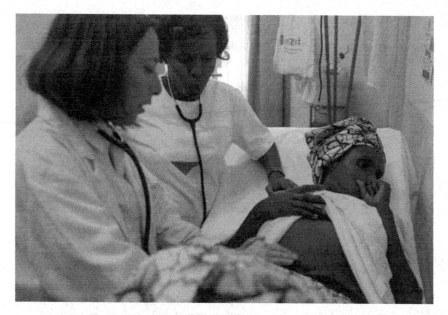

Dr. Mardge Cohen was the Director of the Women and Children's Program at County which provided comprehensive services to women and children with HIV/AIDS. In 2002, in response to women's groups in Rwanda, Mardge and others began a program for women and children in Kigali, Rwanda, based on the lessons learned in Chicago. *(Courtesy Mardge Cohen, MD)*

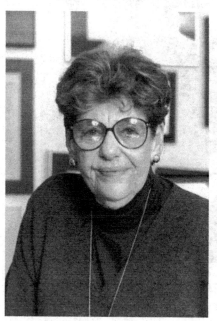

Mrs. Ruth Rothstein was CEO at the Cook County Bureau of Health for fourteen years and a legendary figure in Chicago health care. Prior to coming to County she was credited with keeping an impoverished Mount Sinai Hospital open against all odds. She brought a new era of professional management to the hospital and led the charge for a replacement hospital. *(Courtesy Cook County Health and Hospital System Archives)*

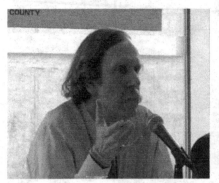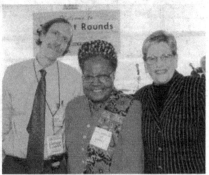

(Left) Dr. Gordy Schiff at "Last Rounds" in September 2002. Gordy's brainchild, "Last Rounds" brought together over four hundred present and former County doctors for an emotional farewell to the "Old Lady on Harrison Street" and a tour of the new hospital. Gordy was the resident intellectual of our group, a health activist and a defender of Cook County Hospital and its patients for more than thirty years. He left County after the budget cuts of 2007 and was recruited to Harvard. (Right) Gordy Schiff, MD, Agnes Lattimer,MD former County Medical Director, and Mrs. Ruth Rothstein, Cook County Bureau of Health Services CEO at "Last Rounds." *(Courtesy Cook County Health and Hospital System Archives)*

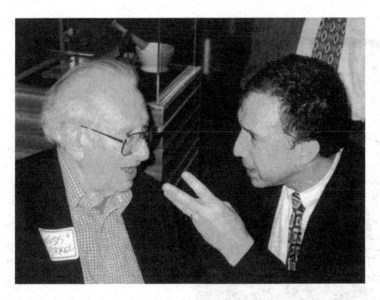

Studs Terkel, the keynote speaker at "Last Rounds," and the author. *(Courtesy Gordon Schiff, MD)*

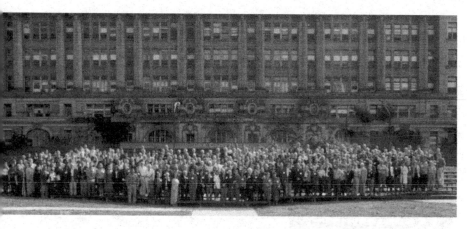

The official "Last Rounds" photo. *(Courtesy Cook County Health and Hospital System Archives)*

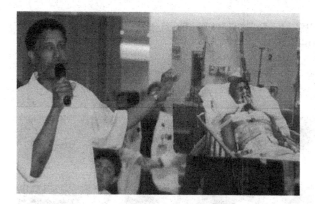

Former West Side Alderman Wallace Davis at "Last Rounds." In the 1970s Davis, a victim of police brutality, spent thirteen months in the County Hospital trauma unit recovering from gunshot wounds. He became an outspoken supporter of County. *(Courtesy Cook County Health and Hospital System Archives)*

Studs Terkel with Dr. Albert Stein, the oldest participant in "Last Rounds." Stein had trained at County in 1935, and was still practicing pediatrics in his nineties. *(Courtesy Cook County Health and Hospital System Archives)*

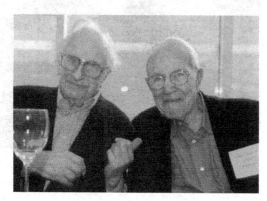

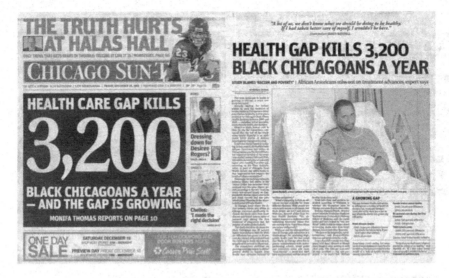

Top: *Chicago Sun-Times* front page article on the racial health disparity in Chicago. Many believe that the failures of the Chicago public health care system contributed to the racial mortality gap. Bottom: Quentin Young with filmmaker Michael Moore, whose film, "Sicko," focused on the failings of our health system. *(Courtesy Health and Medicine Policy Research Group)*

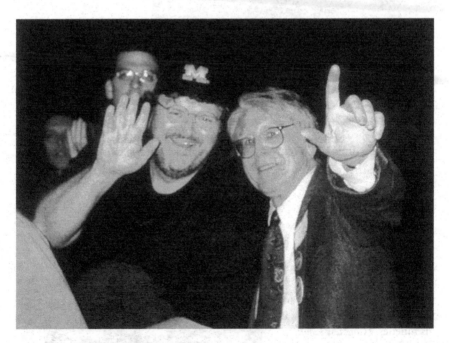

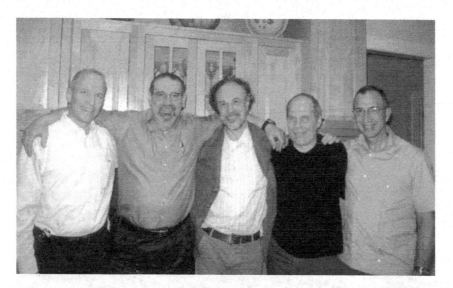

Five of the original "Syracuse Group." From left to right, Stuart Kiken, Barry Abrams, Daniel Brauner, Jim Schlosser and the author, thirty-three years after our internships. *(Courtesy Barry Abrams, MD)*

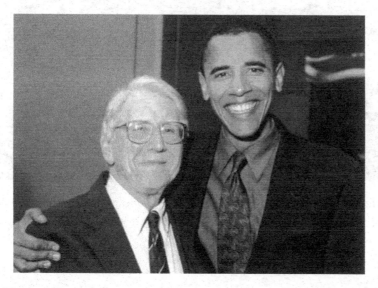

An older Quentin Young, with President Obama. Young is still a health activist into his eighties. Obama supported single-payer health care while a state senator, but abandoned it on the presidential campaign trail. *(Courtesy Health and Medicine Policy Research Group)*

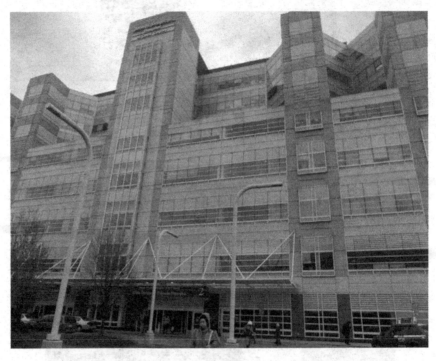

The new John H. Stroger, Jr. Hospital of Cook County, which opened in 2002, eighty-eight years after the old County Hospital was built. *(Courtesy author)*

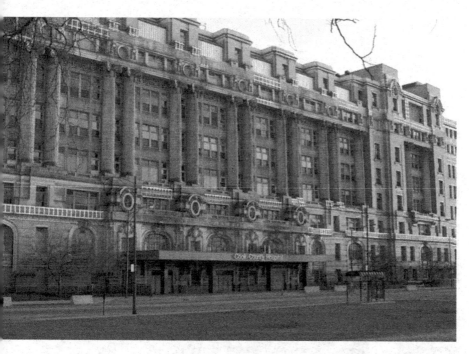

The shuttered old County Hospital in 2010, a silent sentinel to the health care wars in Chicago. *(Courtesy David Goldberg, MD)*

The plaque on the statue at Pasteur Park whose words reflect the mission of the Cook County Health System. *(Courtesy Rush Photo Group)*

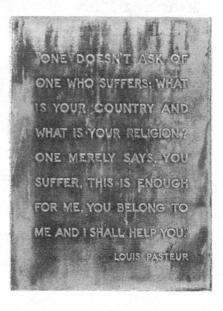

"ONE DOESN'T ASK OF ONE WHO SUFFERS: WHAT IS YOUR COUNTRY AND WHAT IS YOUR RELIGION? ONE MERELY SAYS, YOU SUFFER, THIS IS ENOUGH FOR ME, YOU BELONG TO ME AND I SHALL HELP YOU."

LOUIS PASTEUR

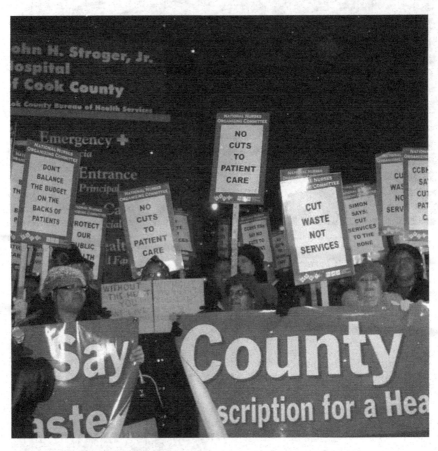

"Plus ça change," a demonstration in front of the John H. Stroger, Jr. Hospital of Cook County protesting the budget cuts of 2007. *(Courtesy author)*

CHAPTER 10

1979–1982: Battle-Worn

By the summer of 1979, in the midst of all of this political activity, crises and tumult, I was on the verge of completing my internship and becoming a second-year resident. A year after travelling from Syracuse to Cook County Hospital, all my medical school friends and I felt a great deal of confidence in our skills. We had arrived at County green and inexperienced and now, a year later, were confident that we could meet just about any clinical challenge placed in front of us. Our political skills had been honed as well, through meetings, rallies and demonstrations. July brought a new batch of interns and we were now the seasoned residents who would show them the ropes. It was trial by fire and we had survived.

I spent the month of July working in the Pediatric Emergency Room at County. The waiting room was packed with crying children and their mothers, who tried to console them. There is nothing scarier than a sick baby, feverish, limp and listless with an infection. I saw the fear in the eyes of the young mothers, who waited hours to see us. The trip to the County Pediatric Emergency Room was daunting. The baby woke up in the middle of the night sick, inconsolable and feverish. The mother touched her lips to the baby's forehead. The forehead was hot, on fire with fever. It's all touch; none of our patients owned a thermometer. She wrapped her baby in a blanket, and woke her other children. They cried in protest. She dressed them and dragged them to the nearest bus stop. The night owl service on the CTA was spotty.

It might take her two or three buses to get to County. Hours passed. For a very sick baby, time mattered. Sometimes, the registration clerks called the nurse when they saw the baby and a nurse ran the languid child back to us, the mother and other children in tow. The moms looked to us in anticipation, though we were not much older than they. We bent over the child who lay lethargic and short-of-breath on the examination table, one of us placed an intravenous line and the other examined the child.

Through exposure to the sheer volume of sick kids, we gained experience. After one especially busy night treating asthma and sewing up lacerations, I staggered into the 8:00 a.m. morning conference with Jim Schlosser, my med school classmate. We were a few minutes late, styrofoam cups of coffee in hand. A group of new interns sat around the table. Like a couple of Vietnam vets, we were battle-scarred old hands. It showed. We had struggled together through medical school, came to County together and now had a year of residency under our belts. The attending physician was teaching the new interns. Our late entry interrupted him. He was a young guy, baby-faced and bald, new to County. He was wearing a Mickey Mouse tie. He tossed a dirty look our way as we pushed open the classroom door and found our seats. His face reddened. Trouble. He stopped his lecture, turned his back on us, then drew a clock onto the blackboard with white chalk:

"Eight o'clock is when Mickey's little hand is on the eight and Mickey's big hand is on the 12," he said in a voice that dripped with condescension as he drew the hands on the clock. His head nodded up and down like a bobble doll.

"You are late for conference."

Jim and I stopped in our tracks, glanced at each other, then back at the young professor. We were primed to address any perceived injustice. This time it was directed at us. We pounced.

"That was so patronizing," Jim said. "How dare you?"

The interns around the conference table stared down at their hands in awkward silence. I wasted no time to pile on, "That's no way to speak to us. Do you know that we have been up all night taking care of patients? This is the last thing we want to hear," I added.

More words were exchanged and the attending, not expecting a double-barreled response from a couple of upstart residents, stammered, turned beet-red and walked out of the conference room. Conference over. We were arrogant (and wrong). We felt as if we had paid our dues. The lines of authority were blurred in those days. Because we were unionized, we functioned almost autonomously from the attending physicians who were less engaged in patient care (Pediatrics was the exception). We were the backbone of the institution. We were leading the fight to keep the hospital open. So our response to attending physicians was sometimes dismissive. Where were they when we needed them?

Upon completion of the internship year, I became a resident. There were three years of an internal medicine residency (four if you were doing it part time as I was) and in the second and third year I had the chance to apply my skills, to apply the knowledge and experience acquired the prior year. But leadership had its challenges.

We were required to provide medical care at the Cook County Jail as part of the residency training. Like much of our other work we were on our own. The Cook County Jail had capacity for about five thousand prisoners, but because of the high arrest rates for blacks and other minorities it had bulged to a point where, on any given day, ten thousand prisoners were housed there. Because the prisoners were all pretrial, they had a constitutional right to free health care. We were it.

We stayed overnight on-call in the jail hospital. Sick patients were brought in from the cell blocks. Rapes. Seizures. Sometimes inmates faked illness to get themselves transferred to the jail ward at County Hospital where the conditions were cushier. Sometimes it was difficult to distinguish the real illnesses from the imagined. One night an old man was brought to the hospital from one of the cell blocks. Dead on arrival. From the looks of him he was in his late sixties. There was not much of a history. He had been arrested by the Chicago police for driving erratically and had been thrown into jail. He had a history of diabetes. On the cell block he had become increasingly confused. The other prisoners had been asking the guards to get him medical attention. He was found dead in his cell. When the inmates on the block learned about his death they refused to eat. They feared the food was contaminated or poisoned. I suspected that the patient had diabetes or a stroke and that he should have been in a hospital instead of jail.

"I have to investigate his death," I told the grim-jawed correctional officer. "Take me to his cell block. I need to speak with the other prisoners and the guards."

"They are not guards. They are officers," he said, a scowl on his face. "Besides, you are not allowed on the cell blocks. I don't have permission."

"This man is dead!" I said. "I need to know why. I am the doctor in charge and I am obligated to conduct an investigation. I have to speak to the other prisoners." I was completely freelancing now, making things up as I went along. The officer relented. He made a few phone calls and we were on our way. The blue-shirted officer had a tight-lipped grimace on his face as he accompanied me on the clanking steel-barred elevator as it clambered past water-stained, paint-peeled floors up to the cell block. It was nighttime and only the dimmed yellow glow of light from the incandescent bulbs lit the eerie way. Another blue-uniformed guard unlocked the door to the cell block with a large metal key and walked me on to the block. A central recreation area was surrounded by a series of small steel-barred cells. As soon as I walked into the block I was mobbed by a group of prisoners who yelled over each other to relay their concerns about the old man's death. I settled the group down and interrogated them one by one about the circumstances of the dead man's short incarceration there. He was sick when he arrived, they reported. Too sick to leave his cell. They tried to get him medical attention but were unable. I concluded that it was not the food but an underlying, undetected disease that caused the man's death. It saddened me to think of this sick old man dying on a County Jail cellblock. Alone. Taken to jail instead of a hospital.

The working conditions at the jail hospital were worse than at County Hospital. We could not get X-rays or blood tests at night at the jail hospital. Pharmaceuticals were in short supply. We had no back up. A group of us convened and we decided that the patient-care conditions were so unacceptable at the jail that we would refuse as a group to provide service there anymore. A work action. We expected a backlash but, instead, the hospital agreed and we were relieved of our duties. Dr. Jack Raba was hired as Medical Director to address the clinical services at the jail. This was the same Dr. Raba who, as House Staff leader during the strike five years earlier, had been jailed for contempt of court. He became a national leader in correctional medicine as a result of his experiences at the Cook County Jail. And he was the only medical director of whom it could be said that he knew the jail inside and out.

Politics crept into the medical care at the hospital. After the County Board seized control of County Hospital in late 1980, the County Board president, George Dunne, imposed a ban on elective abortions at County except if the mother's life was at risk. This ruling had shut down elective abortions at County for years despite the fact that they were legal in the U.S. About 250 pro-choice demonstrators disrupted a County Board meeting to protest the ban, which would not be lifted for over a decade.

This ban would affect one of my patients. One night when I was on call, my team received a young Mexican immigrant woman who had an extremely hyperactive thyroid gland. She had what was called "thyroid storm." Her eyes were bulging, her heart rate rapid and thready. She was sweating profusely and had the characteristic tremors associated with this illness. In addition, she had gone so long without treatment that her liver was enlarged and her heart was in the early stages of failure as evidenced by her swollen ankles, enlarged liver and distended neck veins. Luckily, I had an intern who spoke Spanish and could communicate with her. The treatment of hyperthyroidism included taking medications to slow the heart and block the effect of excess thyroid hormone on the muscles. It also necessitated treatment with radioactive iodine which destroyed the thyroid gland and reduced the production of the excessive thyroid hormone. Unless the woman was pregnant, in which case surgery was the treatment.

Because I knew this patient would be treated with radioactive iodine, I wanted to ensure that she was not pregnant. A fetus exposed to radioactive iodine after twelve weeks of pregnancy could have its thyroid destroyed and be born with cretinism, a form of severe and irreversible mental retardation. The patient refused a pelvic examination because she denied having had sexual intercourse and her urine pregnancy test was negative. I was reassured. Within twenty-four hours she had received the radioactive iodine and we were completing her work-up which included an ultrasound examination of her enlarged liver. I was not prepared for the call I received from the ultrasound lab.

"Dr. Ansell," the physician on the other end of the receiver spoke in the sing-song lilting tones characteristic of the Southern India English dialect, "the liver is fine but when we were examining the liver we saw that she has a 14-week intrauterine pregnancy. Did you know she was pregnant?"

I held the receiver away from my ear in shock and disbelief. Know this? Of course I did not know this. Pregnant? How? We did a urine pregnancy test and it was negative. I learned subsequently that the urine pregnancy tests we used in those days were not reliable after 45 days of pregnancy. Now I had exposed this woman's fetus to a toxic dose of radioactive iodine. A serious medical error. It was my fault, and irreversible. My intern and I spoke to the patient and explained the situation to see what she wanted to do. She was unmarried, and alone in the U.S. She wanted to terminate the pregnancy. This was easier said than done, given the ban on the procedure.

Under the new County policy, we had to prove that the mother's life was at risk. I was on my own. The patient was seriously ill, with heart disease. But was her heart disease a risk to her life? I felt bad for this young woman. An immigrant to Chicago, she spoke no English.

I had screwed up. I should have done a pelvic examination myself. Or sent a more reliable serum pregnancy test rather than rely on the urine test. But it was too late now. I needed a plan. The OB physician was willing to terminate the pregnancy but had to abide by the dictates of the new policy for fear of losing his job. A committee of doctors had to agree.

I called the Chief of Cardiology to evaluate her cardiac risk for pregnancy. Not a likely ally. He was a member of the committee and was a vociferous pro-life proponent. When Dunne had initiated the abortion ban, this doctor publicly applauded the decision. He and I had also clashed in the past about issues in the hospital, so I did not expect any support from him. He examined the patient and declared that while she had heart failure, this posed no risk to her life. I made a desperate appeal to Dr. George Dunea, the chairman of the committee. Australian-born and eccentric, Dr. Dunea was the Chief of Nephrology. He had been at Cook County since the early sixties. He was an excellent clinician with a wry sense of humor. His signature physical characteristic was his hair, a long Brylcreamed, shiny, spiral swirl that sat atop his bald pate like a dollop of whipped cream on a piece of pumpkin pie. I did not know what to expect from him, but he examined the patient, overrode the cardiologist's evaluation and approved the abortion. He stuck his neck out for my patient and I am indebted to him to this day.

Experiences like this, while painful, made me tougher. If I had not hustled on behalf of my patient to get her the procedure, it would not have happened. At County I learned to be relentless in trying to help my patients. This relentlessness was a trait that would be useful later in my career. A woman's right to an abortion had been established seven years earlier by the Supreme Court. We had a patient who needed the procedure and a doctor who was willing to do it. If not for the interference from the Cook County Board into the medical affairs at the hospital, it would not have been necessary to go to such extraordinary lengths to get her treated. County was like this. We often felt we had to perform heroics to get our patients the basic care they deserved.

Those years were rocky at the hospital. The political influence in the affairs of the hospital was palpable. Because of the tumult of 1979, by 1980, many more residents had abandoned County to complete their residencies elsewhere. Those of us who stayed redoubled our efforts to provide the best care we could. From that time on, fewer American-trained students, white or black, joined the training programs at the hospital. The takeover of the hospital by the County Board was accompanied by the influx of patronage employees and cronies of the Democratic Machine. Quentin Young, the Chairman of Medicine at the hospital, tendered his resignation after finding it unbearable to serve under the County Board. Meanwhile, we continued to take care of patients as best we could, while we seethed at the take over of the hospital by the dreaded and hated Democratic Machine. While the independent Governing Commission had its faults, the County Board felt like a foreign occupation. On the national scene, Ronald Reagan had defeated Jimmy Carter and assumed the U.S. presidency with policies that felt antithetical to our beliefs and destructive to our patients. Those of us who stayed did our best on behalf of our patients, despite the feeling that dark days were upon us.

CHAPTER 11

1981: County Will Do This to You

"CODE BLUE, WARD 55, CODE BLUE, WARD 55." The disembodied voice of the switchboard operator on the overhead page announced an impending patient death. Her voice was inflected with about the same enthusiasm as a heavy-lidded CTA bus driver announcing intersections on Chicago's West Side. I was in the main hospital building tending to a patient on Ward 20 when I heard the announcement. I lifted my head to hear the location and noticed the heads of the other interns and residents on the floor rising in kind, as if we were a herd of wildebeest on the Serengeti. A warm rush of adrenaline filled my chest, and the brash of acid born of crummy cafeteria coffee burned my throat. I grabbed my papers and stethoscope. Ward 55. My floor. My patients. Trouble. My heart pounded. I had done this drill before, but it still unnerved me. By then, in my third year of internal medicine residency, I divided the panoply of medical conditions into those I walked to and those which demanded a sprint. This was the latter. A race. Code Blue. Cardiac arrest. Six minutes until brain death—if that long. That's if the code was called when the patient arrested. But who knew how long the patient had lain there before a nurse noticed?

I thought back to my early days at County three years before. On Ward 24 during the first week of my internship in July 1978, I walked by a cubicle on my way to lunch and saw an old woman sitting on her chair, feet splayed and her head tilted back, eyes closed, her mouth wide open with tongue hanging out in the fashion of sleeping dogs and old people. The "q"-sign. All medical students learned it: the tongue resembles the curly tail of a "q"; the open mouth the circle. An old person sleeping. Or dead. The thought passed my mind as my stomach rumbled. Now, as a senior resident, I knew better to trust my instincts. County taught you that. Hadn't I noticed her in the same position when I came in this morning? I was tempted to walk in and check. But she wasn't my patient and I was hungry. I walked the ten minutes to the cafeteria, ambled through the line and was eating when the call for a Code Blue was announced. Ward 24. I knew it was she. I ran back. Two city blocks. Too long. County was designed for failure. It was the old lady. Not asleep. Dead in her chair, "q"-sign and all frozen permanently on her face. She was surrounded by doctors and nurses who tried to revive her. Not this time. At least forty minutes had passed since I first walked by on my way to the cafeteria. Maybe more. My first Code at County.

This case replayed in my head in slow-motion, like a World War II newsreel, whenever I responded to a Code Blue. I recalled that old lady as I ran out of Ward 20 on my way to Ward 55. I sprinted the forty-yard dash, papers flapping, while I maintained a tight grip on my stethoscope against the clipboard, past the nursing station, around the corner to the stairwell, then down the two flights to the main lobby two steps at a time, a long run down the cavernous hallway, a sharp left before the information desk with the lone security guard, a stone-faced sphinx nursing a coffee and reading the *Sun-Times*. I ran through the double wooden doors with chicken wire glass windows into the Emergency Room waiting room already stacked with people; standing room only at 8:00 a.m. Past the triage desks, I ignored the pleas and outreached arms of patients who had probably waited for hours if not days, like beggars in a Mumbai market. They beseeched me as I ran by, calling, "Doctor, doctor!"

I pushed through the emergency room doors, past the "No Admittance" sign. I skirted nurses and the patients in cloth hospital gowns, who lay moaning on stretchers lined up like salmon at Pike's Market. At one time, I might have been aghast at the sight of this suffering, but now, three years into my training, my nerve endings had been anesthetized. I felt nothing. I ran through the treatment area and out another set of doors to the ambulance-receiving area, past the two Chicago cops who slouched at the Chicago Police Department station located at the back entrance of the Emergency Department, indifferent to the chaos around them. I straight-armed one of the doors that led to the ambulance bay, jumped down four feet to the tarmac. The icy winter chill slapped me across my face and choked me with my first breath of the icy air. Now for the 25 yard sprint from the ambulance bay to the Medical A Building, a yellow brick building, squat and nondescript, that sat facing Wood Street, behind the main hospital.

I ran into the elevator lobby through A Building's steel door, barely wide enough for a stretcher to pass. I checked if either of the two elevators was there (they never were when you needed them), punched the elevator button with my closed fist in frustration and ran up the stairs, two by two, sucking mouthfuls of air for five flights to Ward 55.

I shoved open the door to the ward and spotted the crowd of nurses and the red crash cart. Sweat poured down my arms. My glasses were fogged over with condensation. Many of the patients here had been admitted over the past month by my team.

As a senior resident, I was at the mercy of my two interns, first-year trainees. There were just too many patients to manage by myself. We all knew the good ones and the bad ones. The first-year residents were ranked like March Madness college teams in an office pool. We rated them just as our seniors had rated us when we were interns. Sometimes if we sweet-talked the scheduler in the Department of Medicine we got the interns we wanted on our team. And sometimes the weak ones were paired with a strong resident for the sake of the patients.

B.T. was one of my interns, a weak doctor, and two weeks into the rotation he was making mistakes and killing patients. He was a foreign-trained American (almost always a red flag) who spent a large part of the 1970s as a pot-smoking college drop-out. The Indians, Pakistanis and Middle Easterners were generally better trained than

Americans who trained abroad. Now, at age 35 or 36, he had matriculated from an Italian medical school and landed a County internship—not too difficult if you were an American and spoke English, especially given the recent exodus of doctors. He looked like a college professor with his balding pate, graying temples and beard, and we all wanted to believe that behind those thoughtful eyes and well-chosen words was the mind of a great physician. But he was shaky. One night on-call, early in the rotation, before I was on to him, he let a patient die, out of ignorance.

It was one of those nights. Patients rolled in one after another. I could not keep up. In resident parlance, we were getting "smashed." Given the shakiness of nursing coverage at the hospital, the lives of the patients often depended on the strength of our doctors to fill in the gaps. B.T. presented a case to me of a small older woman with a urinary tract infection whom he said was doing well. I asked him to check her lab tests and call me if anything was wrong. I never heard from him and assumed everything was fine. Wrong. Just before dawn, I found her on the unit, in a bed, dead. When I checked her labs to see what had gone wrong, I noticed that her blood test showed her bicarbonate level was dangerously low, something that signified acid had built up in the blood, a very bad sign in the presence of an infection. She needed to be in the Intensive Care Unit. My intern had missed it, and the patient died. I hadn't trusted him since that incident. So when I saw the crowd of nurses encircling the patient's bed on Ward 55, my heart sank when I realized that the patient the nurses were attending belonged to my Italian-trained intern.

I gulped as I sprinted the last fifty feet to the patient's bedside. Six minutes had passed since I left the other building. A Filipino nurse yelled, "Doc, he has no pulse!" This was not supposed to happen. The patient was admitted with pneumonia and was ready to go home. Now we struggled to revive him.

"What happened?" I asked.

"We came to give him his meds, and he was unresponsive, so we called a Code Blue."

I listened to his chest with my stethoscope and felt for a carotid pulse by placing my fingers along the side of his throat. The fetid smell of death wafted into my nose from his open mouth. "No pulse!" I confirmed. "Begin CPR." I clasped my hands together. My fingers interlocked, and I leaned over the patient, my arms straight. I placed the heel of my left hand in the center of his lifeless sternum and began chest compressions, using the weight of my body to pump his heart. "One and two and three and four and. . ." I compressed in the rhythm I was taught in a class long ago. The patient grunted as my compressions forced air out of his glottis. Another resident ran to the head of the bed and ventilated him with an ambu bag, a type of air pump used to breathe for a patient.

"What's the rhythm?" I asked.

"V fib," yelled a nurse.

"Defibrillator," I said. I grabbed the defibrillator paddles. "Step back," I said. I charged the defibrillator, and the air filled with a high-pitched whine as the electrical charge pulsated toward the paddles. I placed the defibrillator paddles on the left side of his chest, made sure my body was not touching any metal on the bed, and pushed the buttons on the paddle, delivering the 200 millivolts to the patient's chest. He jumped like a rag doll with the jolt.

"Rhythm?" I inquired. The needle on the EKG machine quivered irregularly as yards of EKG paper spilled onto the floor. "Still V fib, doc. No pulse."

"Continue CPR," I commanded. I resumed chest compressions. I felt a crack as the force of my weight broke a rib. A momentary wave of nausea threatened.

"Give me the defibrillator at 400 millivolts," I asked. I went through the routine and shock again. His lifeless body jumped with the electric jolt, then plopped back into the bed. "Still V fib, no pulse. Continue CPR."

"Epi, 1/10000 IV, 2 amps of bicarb, IV, get a blood gas. Do we have a good line?" I asked.

Another resident grabbed the patient's chart and read through it. "He's a diabetic; he got a big dose of insulin last night."

My intern must have ordered too much insulin. "Check a sugar!" I asked.

A medical student tied a tourniquet around the patient's wrist, drew a tube of blood, and ran it down to the laboratory in the ICU five flights below.

"Give Dextrose 50, 2 amps." How could I have forgotten such a basic step? A rookie error. Insulin, if given in too high a dose, caused the blood sugar to fall so low that the patient could become unresponsive and even go into cardiac arrest. I should have given him a lifesaving sugar solution right when I arrived at his bedside. I still kick myself today about forgetting this basic step.

We shocked him again and coaxed a weak pulse to return. His blood sugar rose—low, too low for life. We gave more sugar solution. The intensive care team arrived and transferred the patient to the ICU. Almost thirty minutes had passed since the original call. If he woke up at all, his brain would be jello. An avoidable error. On my watch.

I sat, drained, demoralized and spent, shoulders slumped, head down, on the patient's now empty bed as the nurses picked up strips of EKG paper and empty syringes from the floor. The winter morning sun poured in through the east-facing windows as if to mock my gloom. I had a full day of rounding ahead of me and was already behind. A patient was dead or close to it. Tomorrow—on-call again. A familiar feeling of dread rose from my gut—a feeling that I had experienced many times before during my training. That I was not a good enough doctor yet. All of the fights we had endured, all the demonstrations and rallies we had attended to ensure the survival of the hospital fell to the wayside when a patient got ill or suffered a complication. In the end it was about the patients and when I fell short, I beat myself up about it. We all did. But just as soon as the feeling of doubt presented itself, I had to let it go. No time for it. I summoned my strength, picked up my clipboard full of patients' notes, and shuffled off the floor to begin rounds with my team.

CHAPTER 12

1983–1986: Amateur Sociologists

THE SHRILL RING OF THE PHONE on the back counter of the County Emergency Room pierced the din of the busy night. I was a senior resident in the County Emergency Room for my last time. I was stationed in the "center" of the Emergency Room; the main stage. By now I was very experienced. Gone were the rookie jitters and the anxieties of being in charge of the ER by myself. I was a veteran. Amazed by what the last few years of training had done for my confidence and skills, I picked up the receiver.

"Hello, this is Dr Ansell, Cook County Emergency."

"Yeah, this is the Emergency Room at University of XXX. We would like to transfer a patient to you."

I knew the routine. I had received these calls many times.

County Hospital was the hospital of last resort for the undesirable. It was the hospital for black people, for immigrants and the mentally ill. Most of all it was the hospital for the uninsured. And the reigning practice at other hospitals in the Chicago area was to transfer uninsured patients to County. I do not remember being formally taught about this aspect of the job as a medical resident in the Emergency Room. It was passed down from resident to resident. An oral tradition. Pick up the phone and accept the patient.

"What's wrong with the patient?" I asked. I knew from experience that the answer could be anything. Sometimes it was a patient with a gunshot wound to the head on a ventilator. Other times it was a patient with pneumonia. A heart attack. Or a woman in the final stages of labor. Sometimes they didn't tell the truth. It did not matter. We accepted them all.

"What's the reason for transfer?" I asked.

"No insurance," said the doctor on the phone. "Okay," I said, "send 'em."

Next to the phone was a clipboard filled with transfer forms on which we were supposed to document the hospital calling, the name and condition of the patient, the diagnosis and the reason for transfer. The most common reason cited for the transfer to County was that the patient had "no insurance."

Something happened with transfers to County in the early 1980s that caught our attention. The phone in the back of the Emergency Room began to ring more frequently. Hospitals from around the county called to transfer patients to us more often. Ambulances from other hospitals unloaded patients on stretchers with increasing frequency at the back door of the Emergency Room. The number of transfers to County increased from 100 each month in the late 1970s to over 600 each month by the early 1980s. The major reason for these transfers was the growing number of uninsured in the Chicago area and the decision by the State of Illinois to limit the payment for those patients on Public Aid to $500 per hospitalization. But this was not just a Chicago phenomenon; the number of transfers to public hospitals were on the rise all around the United States. Factory closings during the previous two decades had left thousands of workers either jobless or in jobs without health-care benefits. Of course, minorities and the urban working poor were disproportionately affected. These were the Reagan years and we were feeling the disastrous impact of Reaganomics on inner city Chicago. There was no "Morning in America" when it came to health care in Chicago. Hospitals were struggling to stay afloat with the rising tide of the uninsured. Emergency Room visits were up. In Chicago, fourteen hospitals were shuttered in the 1980s for financial reasons.

The remaining hospitals developed policies to keep uninsured patients out. They performed a financial screen, called a "wallet biopsy" by cynics, when patients came to the emergency room. They limited the care they provided if patients were not adequately insured. If a patient needed hospitalization, he or she was transferred to Cook County. The phenomenon came to be called "patient dumping." These patients were often very sick, sometimes critically ill. Some died or suffered irreversible complications as a result. But dumping was accepted medical practice across the United States, and rarely questioned. A group of us, all of whom had been on the receiving end of these calls, met to discuss the problem. "We should do something about this."

I had spent the last seven years learning to become a doctor. It had taken much of my focus and energy. We had been fighting for the life of the hospital as well. These transfers of uninsured patients to the hospital had been going on for ages. It was just the way things worked in Chicago. No one questioned it. But the more we talked about this routine practice, the more appalled we became. It was one thing for a sick patient to come directly to the Cook County Emergency Room for treatment. We had to take care of these patients. But if a sick patient showed up at another hospital, shouldn't that hospital have the same obligation to treat that patient if they had the capacity? We had seen patients with illnesses whose treatment was delayed or deferred because they had no insurance, sometimes with devastating consequences. Patients who arrived in cardiac arrest, or dead. But no one would listen to a bunch of County Hospital docs who complained about injustice. We needed to document the problem in meticulous detail and publish the results.

A colleague, Bob Schiff, led the study. Jim Schlosser, my friend from medical school, now working in the County Emergency Room, joined with another Emergency Room colleague. I was completing a Chief Residency, an extra residency year, and joined the group. We recruited an epidemiologist, Steven Whitman, to help with the analysis and began to meet every week to strategize. We decided to track the clinical outcomes of 500 consecutive patients who were transferred to County from other hospitals. That was about three weeks worth of patients. For three weeks, one of us went to the Emergency Room each day to see which patients had been transferred. We collected all the records, including the transfer forms that were filled out by the residents on the prior day's shift. We also interviewed the patients to find out what they had been told at the other hospital about the reason for transfer. We then reviewed all of the patients' charts.

It was one thing to be on the receiving end of a few phone calls each shift as a resident in the Emergency Room. It was another to track 500 of these patients and follow what actually happened to them. The nature of the calls and the patient outcomes were horrifying. Patients were transferred on ventilators, with gunshot wounds, in active labor. I remember one transferred patient, in the terminal part of labor, a breech delivery, the baby's foot in the vagina, the woman's cervix fully dilated. She was transferred to County because she had "no insurance." I had been told by obstetricians at County of women who died in the County Emergency Room while delivering babies after transfer. These lives could have been saved if they had received appropriate care at the transferring hospital. It was a legal form of battery, manslaughter or worse and violated the most basic precepts of medicine, "First, do no harm." And these hospitals transferred the patients with complete impunity.

The results of our study were shocking. Over twenty percent of the transferred patients ended up in a medical Intensive Care Unit; of these, nine percent died. Many were in unstable medical condition at the time of transfer. And almost none of the patients gave consent for transfer. In fact, the doctors at the transferring hospital often lied to the patients about the reason for transfer. The patients were often told they were being sent to Cook County because the transferring hospital had no beds. The reason given to the doctors at Cook County for transfer was usually "no insurance."

News of our study traveled around the hospital. Jim Schlosser, who during this period became the Director of the Cook County Emergency Department, was concerned about the negative repercussions of our work. A smoldering conflict began to divide us. Jim was getting pushback from some physicians and senior administrators that our study was dangerous for the hospital. There was a group of trauma surgeons who strongly believed that County should be accepting these patients in transfer regardless of their initial condition because they would get better treatment at County than at community hospitals. They were trying to establish a regional trauma network in Chicago which would require trauma patients to come to the nearest trauma center, bypassing the community hospitals. If our study resulted in ending transfers to Cook County Hospital, their dreams of a regional trauma network might be threatened. "How could we criticize hospitals for transferring uninsured patients?" others asked. "Isn't this what public hospitals are for?" Jim voiced their concerns.

Bob Schiff and I disagreed. Most of the transferred patients had common medical conditions: pneumonia; women in active labor; conditions that could be treated at almost any hospital. Transfer just delayed treatment, for financial, not clinical, reasons. It was unconscionable. Nothing in our study negated the importance of trauma networks. But the ideological battle lines had been drawn. The bitterness around this debate insinuated itself into our group. Our meetings grew more contentious.

The second floor of Fantus Clinic had a row of windowless offices. We sat clustered in a tight circle of chairs between desks cluttered with papers as we debated the implications of our study. I had borrowed one of the first commercial personal computers, a K-Pro, from Gordy Schiff, Bob's brother, to write the first drafts of the paper. I worked at night at my dining room table in our third floor walk-up apartment while my wife Paula and our young son slept.

While we agreed on the facts of the paper, we brawled over words. Bob and I insisted on including the words "patient dumping" in our title and in the discussion of our results. We did not want to mince words. "Dumping" was a powerful and accurate depiction of the process. Jim thought the words were inflammatory, pejorative and political and wanted to call dumping "economic transfers." Bob and I thought this was a cop out. The other physician sided with Jim. We were split down the middle. We clashed for weeks. Voices escalated and tempers flared. Shouts erupted in the closed office and the conflict spilled out into the hallways. Our colleagues in the adjacent offices would see us after these marathon battles and give us inquisitive looks. The four of us had started out together on the same page and now the differences had become personal and sometimes antagonistic.

Jim and I had been close friends for eleven years, since the first year of medical school in 1974. So much in common—medical school and late-night talks on the couch of our house in Syracuse. We shared some of the same doubts about medicine during the first two years of medical school. We came together to train at County. We had fought together for the survival of the hospital. Before we worked on the patient dumping problem we had always been on the same side of so many issues. Now there was a wedge between us. The ER Director job was an important administrative job in the hospital and it was a testimony to Jim's administrative skills that he was given this job at such a young age. I remember noticing Jim make the personal transition from a gray-eyed, blond-haired, pony-tailed resident into a well-dressed, professional-looking, white-coated attending physician. He felt a different level of obligation to the institutional leadership than Bob and I, and must have been under a lot of pressure because of the study. As I reflect back on that time, I am sure Jim felt betrayed by my lack of support for him. In the end, after weeks of heated arguments and an inability to reach consensus, we agreed to a compromise that was accepted more out of weariness than principle. In the discussion section of the paper appear these well-crafted words: "these economic transfers also known as patient dumping." We split the differences between us down the middle.

Our paper, "Transfers to a Public Hospital," was published by the *New England Journal of Medicine* in 1986, and was one of the first articles to depict the negative health outcomes associated with patient dumping in a large city in the U.S. None of us had done research before nor ever written a paper. We had few mentors to advise us and were not prepared for the local and national response to our paper's release.

In anticipation of the publication of the paper we prepared a press release and organized a press conference. The County public relations office was forbidden to work with us. We were on our own. The hospital was so concerned about the results of our study that, to our surprise, they held a competing press conference in another room to criticize our paper. This was the most important study to come from Cook County Hospital in the last fifty years and we were pariahs in our own institution. The practice of patient dumping had been the status quo in Cook County for the last hundred years and our paper threatened to end it. The private hospitals had reasons to want the practice to continue. Even George Dunne, the County Board President, criticized the study and called us a bunch of "amateur sociologists."

Despite the fierce local opposition, the response to our article was electric. Across the country, the tragedy of patient dumping in the midst of the Reagan era's prosperity was viewed as an indictment of the U.S. health care system. The *Chicago Tribune* and the *Wall Street Journal* featured the story on their front pages. *Nightline* and the *McNeil-Lehrer Report* each did television segments on the problem. We wrote a piece for *USA Today* and were interviewed by other media outlets. The press hounded us for interviews for months after the publication.

Just as things began to return to normal, we received a phone call from Congressional staffers. They asked us to come to Washington to testify before the House Committee on Inter-Governmental Affairs. I flew to Washington to give the testimony. Before the testimony, we had many conversations with senior staff who were trying to craft potential legislative solutions.

The room where I was to testify was in the Sam Rayburn Building on Capitol Hill. It was cavernous, with oversized windows that overlooked the boulevard outside. The congressmen and staff sat on a raised dais at the front. I sat at a rectangular, government-standard, witness table in the front of the room. I stated my name, raised my right hand and swore to tell the truth. My voice quavered as I read from my two-page testimony that outlined the findings of our study and suggested specific policy changes. Emergency treatment at a hospital should include treatment available in a hospital beyond an Emergency Room that was within the capabilities of a hospital. Hospitals should be required to treat patients requiring emergency care first and then check insurance status later rather than the other way around. Patients should be informed that they have a right to emergency treatment. Before transferring a patient to another hospital, the patients should give informed consent that would include the risks of being transferred and should only be transferred for services not available at the transferring hospital. There should be large fines for violating these rules. The finish was anticlimactic. No one asked any questions. I walked out of the Capitol and caught the next flight home.

We later learned that our study and other reports of patient dumping around the country led to legislative changes that make the interhospital transfer of uninsured patients more difficult. The Emergency Medical Treatment and Active Labor Act passed Congress in 1986 and encoded most of our recommendations into law. Since then, it has been a violation of federal law to transfer a patient without first performing a screening medical examination which might include testing and treatment available outside the emergency department. Patients could only be transferred with consent and for medical reasons. Violations of the law could lead to fines of up to $250,000 and loss of Medicare funding for the hospital. The U.S. Congress also expanded the Medicaid program, allowing all uninsured pregnant women to be presumptively covered by the government insurance program so hospitals and doctors could get paid. Our study, born from outrage, had contributed to the regulation of the most egregious forms of patient dumping in the U.S. The numbers of uninsured patients transferred to County Hospital dropped, almost overnight. Not bad for a bunch of amateur sociologists.

CHAPTER 13

1983: Moving On

I SAT ON THE CHAIR in front of an oversized desk. The large walnut conference table to my left, where morning report was held, looked forlorn without the usual complement of residents and attending physicians sitting around it to discuss cases. The bookshelves were filled with medical textbooks and bound journals, lined up like soldiers, not one out of place. The room was ice cold. The air conditioner in the corner window blasted arctic air across the room.

The desk in front of me was covered with piles of journal articles. Behind the desk sat Dr. O, the Chairman of Medicine. His brow was furrowed. He was reading an article. He did not acknowledge my presence. His modus operandi. I did not take this personally. He was like this to almost everyone. Avuncular and quirky, Dr. Quentin Young, my former chairman, left County Hospital shortly after the County Board took over from the Governing Commission. His replacement, Dr. O., was a brilliant physician, but an unhappy man and glacier cold. "He lacked the milk of human kindness," one of his colleagues said of him. Dr. O did not suffer fools. He was a master of psychological intimidation whose icy stares and long silences could cast a pall on even the most fearless of us. I gritted my teeth and braced myself every time we met. Today, I squirmed in my seat and waited to be recognized. I was at a disadvantage. I needed something from him. A job. My residency was about to end and I wanted to stay at County. He looked up from his article, eyebrows raised in query, his hooded eyes, which made him look reptilian, scanned me from head to toe. A prominent temporal vein snaked along his temples.

I had reasons to be concerned about his response to my job inquiry. I had been outspoken and willing to express my disagreements with Dr. O. We clashed on occasion. I did not think he liked me much. But it was hard to tell with him. One recent confrontation stood out. I had organized a meeting between the residents and him. To say it had not gone well would be a serious understatement. Dr. O had recently appointed one of the attending physicians to be departmental vice chairman. None of us wanted this doctor to be in this position of authority.

I arranged the meeting to give Dr. O our feedback. Dr. O did not like to receive feedback. Before the meeting, all the residents expressed trepidation about speaking first. Dr. O had a sharp tongue and a reputation for ripping young residents to shreds. I made a deal with the residents. "Okay, I'll start and then you need to jump right in behind me. All right? You've got my back?" They all agreed. The meeting was at the end of the day in a small conference room. We sat and waited for the showdown. The dim ceiling light gave the room a yellowish hue. The staccato rhythm of Dr. O's footsteps ricocheted off the walls of the room and proclaimed his arrival. A scowl was plastered to his face. He was wearing a three-piece suit. In contrast, we were a scruffy and ill-kempt bunch. He sat crossed-armed. "Well?" he said and turned his laser gaze on me. I stammered my way through the explanation for the meeting and asked him to reconsider his choice for vice chair. I knew what would happen next.

He ripped into me like a pit bull into a piece of fresh meat. "How dare you question my pick for vice chair," he said. "It's absolutely none of your business." I was the sacrificial lamb. Just as we had planned. Chopped, chewed, digested and spat out. A propitious start. We had him where we wanted him. Now, here came the reinforcements. Right? All the other residents who promised me they would speak up? Wrong. "Speak up fellow residents," I thought, "speak up." Silence. Not one peep from the twenty-five other residents in the room. "Does anyone else have anything to say?" Dr. O said. "No one?" he asked again, while eyeing all the residents in the room. The rest of the residents hung their heads, careful not to make eye contact. "Then I'll be leaving." He shoved his chair aside and shot me a scorching glance. The chair gave a metallic screech as he got up and walked out.

So it was with some trepidation that I sat across the desk from him again. On the other hand, I had been a Chief Resident under Dr. O. and he seemed to respect me. Dr. O had an encyclopedic knowledge of medicine and liked to show it off. As chief residents, we held weekly clinical pathological conferences. These conferences were the highlight of the training program, an old County tradition dating back a hundred years. They were held in the old autopsy amphitheatre in the Hektoen Laboratory Building across Wood Street from the hospital. The amphitheatre was like the ones pictured in paintings of autopsies in the 19th century. A stainless steel autopsy table commanded the middle of the room. Semi-circular rows of wooden benches rose up from the floor and hugged the curved wall. An aroma of formaldehyde, used to preserve body parts, wafted through the air. Students, residents and attending physicians were packed into the benches and along the walls. The most popular teaching conference at County for the last hundred years. The chief resident's job was to pick apart a case that was presented to the audience, piece by piece, in bite-size segments. It ended with a review of the pathological findings. Each case was like a detective whodunit with the chief resident, like Perry Mason in a courtroom, asking questions from the audience who attempted to solve the puzzle. The cases were generally stumpers and few in the crowd guessed the diagnosis, until Dr. O became department chairman. Each week at the end of the case and right before the pathologist presented the findings, Dr. O spoke. He wove the various elements of the case together and made a diagnosis. He was always right. It was uncanny, Sherlock Holmesian, always the smartest doctor in the room. Naturally, we were suspicious.

We kept our files for the conference in the chief resident office down from Dr. O's office. The cases were closely held secrets. No one knew the answer except the Chief Resident until the pathologist revealed the diagnosis. But, if you really wanted to know the details of the case, you could sneak into the chief resident office, find the file of the chief resident who was leading the next week's conference and read through it. We suspected that Dr. O might have been discovering the details of our cases in advance. Once I kept the case materials at home. To mask the case from discovery, on the poster announcing the conference, I called the case, "A Man with Chwe-Chwe-Chwe." The patient had sickle cell anemia and died. I used the obscure West African name for the disease, "chwe-chwe-chwe," to avoid discovery. A few days before the conference, I received a call from the medical librarian asking me what the title meant. Dr. O had called her and she needed to get back to him with an answer. We were an anti-authoritarian and suspicious bunch, so we could be accused of paranoia. In fairness to Dr. O he was extremely well-read, a brilliant doctor, so he needed no props to solve a difficult medical brainteaser. Regardless, Dr. O did not endear himself to us and the feeling was mutual.

"I'd like to stay on at County, Dr. O. Are there any positions?" I asked. My original plan was to go back east after residency, but I decided that I wanted to stay on. There was more work to do. To my surprise, Dr. O was friendly and supportive of my desire to stay and join the Division of General Medicine and Primary Care. Dr. O had created the new Division in the Department of Medicine to provide a home for doctors like me who were interested in the field of primary care. Primary Care divisions were a new phenomenon at teaching hospitals in the United States in the early 1980s. And Dr O's foresight created one of the best in the country. We were not the easiest group of doctors to manage. To his credit, he maintained an arm's length relationship with us. In the long run his lack of comfort with us allowed our group to develop a robust set of skills and programs that might not have happened if he had supported us more.

There were initially ten of us in the Division of General Medicine/Primary Care in 1983. Except for one black physician, Dr. Cynthia Watson, all the rest of us were young white physicians. Eventually, the number would grow to fifty and become more diverse. Each of the original group had finished residency training within the past few years at County. We had fought for the survival of the hospital. We were full of ideas on how to improve it. We believed ourselves to be best suited to train the next generation of physicians on the wards at Cook County Hospital. And we were going to do it differently. We would see every inpatient, write notes, hold teaching conferences and provide more support than we ever received during our training. Together, we helped define the future of primary care at Cook County for the next thirty years. Of the original ten young doctors in the fledgling Division of General Medicine in 1983, all went on to have important careers in medicine. One became a national expert on quality and patient safety. Some went off to run successful practices. One ran for alderman as the first openly gay candidate in Chicago. Three physicians became national leaders in the care of patients with HIV infection. Others became experts in the fields of preventive medicine, primary care, adolescent medicine, international health, teaching primary care, and correctional medicine.

We had much in common. We all believed in the importance of universal health care. The leading proponents of single-payer health care in the U.S. had all worked in public hospitals. You could not work at County in those years and think that the U.S. had a fair or functional system of health care, that this was the best this country could do. We believed that health care was a human right. That racism in American society contributed to health inequity. I was excited to join the group. Among the members were the young physicians who had recruited us to come to County from Syracuse, just four years before: Mardge Cohen and Gordy Schiff. Sometimes we fought like cats and dogs. It was inevitable with such a dynamic and passionate group of doctors. Mardge and I had a couple of fur-flying screaming matches over some long-forgotten difference of opinion. Now thirty years later, I have only affectionate memories of that period.

I started my new job after a grueling nine-year period of training: med school, residency, the battles for the survival of the hospital.

I had survived the difficulties that training on the front lines at a place like County presented to me. And I learned a lot about being a doctor. With no more night call, I could breathe a bit. I made a vow to myself. There was so much about the way we treated patients at County that disturbed me. If I stayed on, I had to do something more than practice hospital-based medicine, taking care of end-stage neglected disease. Our patients needed good primary care services. They needed preventive care. I decided that on the cusp of my career I would pursue work in preventive medicine.

I was a simmering cauldron of conflicted emotions. With time to reflect, I realized that the last four years had been more than just a residency training program. Though I had learned to be a good doctor, I had also been a witness to a health-care system in crisis. I had witnessed the destructive corrosion that racism and poverty wrought on the hospital and patients. Where life and death depended on whether or not you had health insurance and on the color of your skin. I had a front row seat to the conflict about fairness in health in America. A war for health equity. From my vantage point, in 1983, the good guys were losing.

In the summer of 1983, a group of us rented a cottage in Union Pier, Michigan, a beach resort an hour away from Chicago. About twenty of us, a mixed-race group of doctors, nurses, and clerks from County, were swimming and lounging on the beach. Paula and I were there with our son. A white home owner threatened to call the police if we did not move from the beach in front of his home. A racist? Or maybe just an asshole. I snapped. A wave of anger overcame me, a hot blast of rage that rose from my belly to my mouth. It was as if the home owner's threat triggered a trip-wire reaction that lay dormant. I was ready for a fight. Red-faced, I went jaw to jaw with the owner and dared him to call the cops. He did. I needed to be restrained by others in the group who yanked me away, as the blue waters of Lake Michigan lapped the white sandy shoreline behind us. The black people in the group were unfazed. They were used to this. Just move, do not make a scene. My physician colleagues looked askance at me, shocked at my outburst. I realized years later that this event had tapped into an internal cauldron of frustration and rage that I had carried around with me. What I had witnessed during my training at County reinforced beliefs that I had held since childhood about the scale of injustice in the world. I had made it through residency, though not unscathed. I was not proud of that moment. My confrontation on the beach triggered feelings that I had kept buried during the last few years. There was more work to be done now that I was an attending physician. I vowed to keep my emotions under control so I could be effective.

CHAPTER 14

Working Against the Odds

THE HIGH-PITCHED BEEPING of my pager pierced the still of the early morning air. My heart rate increased in a Pavlovian response that harkened back to my days as a resident when the beeping often presaged a patient in trouble. It was as if the pager was hardwired to my nervous system. At the screech of a beep beep beep I was wide-eyed, alert and ready to go. Our pagers represented a fragile gossamer of a lifeline between our patients and us. We had no answering service or secretaries to take messages. We were the answering service. Many of us kept our pagers on and at our sides day and night in case a patient needed us. Thirty years later this habit was still hardwired. But today this was not a patient calling.

I unclipped the gray card-deck-sized Motorola pager from my belt and held it about eight inches from my eyes. I pressed the rectangular black button on the top and squinted to view the call back phone number in the dim backlit display. In 1983, these were stone age pagers; clunkers, ready for an exhibit at the Smithsonian, or the trash heap. I recognized the number. Uh-oh. My eyes widened. It was the medical director's office. "Trouble," I grimaced as I scurried to find an available phone.

"This is Dr. Ansell answering a page," I said when the secretary to the medical director answered the phone.

"Good morning, Dr. Ansell. Dr. Brown wants to see you right away."

When I decided to stay at County, I began to have discussions with another member of the General Medicine Division, Arthur Hoffman, about working in prevention and early detection. Arthur was convinced that in order to transform care at County we had to develop preventive medicine programs for our patients and use public health methods to recruit and educate them. I agreed. I wanted a job for myself that allowed me to balance prevention and early detection with the cold realities of the job of an attending physician at County, which mostly focused on sick hospitalized patients with late stage disease. Arthur had started a preventive medicine program in the General Medicine clinic for colorectal cancer detection. He suggested that I focus on breast cancer screening.

In 1977, the first randomized controlled trial on the use of mammography as a screening tool was published and showed that women who receive mammography screening had a twenty to thirty percent reduction in mortality from breast cancer. By 1983, breast cancer screening among white women was becoming more prevalent in the U.S. But at County, a chart review showed that only two percent of all women had received a screening mammogram. At the time, neither the doctors nor the patients at County knew much about the benefits of screening. I read all the papers I could find on the subject. But it was impossible to begin a new program at County without some personnel, and there was no way for a peon like me to get the County Hospital bureaucracy to approve new positions in their annual budget request. Arthur and I decided that we could get the program going if we just had two nurses. But it was an uphill climb. Even if we could convince the County Hospital to include these two new nursing positions in the annual budget request, they might never be approved by the finance committee of the County Board downtown unless one of the Machine politicians wanted them. It was how the game was played.

A long shot, but we had an ace in the hole. Pure luck. There was a new County Commissioner, an independent Democrat, who was also a breast cancer survivor. She agreed to help. If the two nursing positions included in the hospital budget were removed by the politicians downtown, she would make a motion from the floor of the County Board to have them reinstated. Arthur and I knew her administrative aide and he worked behind the scenes to make this happen. But the positions for the two nurses could not be put into the budget without a request from the hospital. The request had to come from the Chairman of the Department of Medicine, and Dr. O refused to include them in his budget request. And the medical director, Dr. Rowine Brown, refused to answer calls from Arthur to meet. We were too low on the feeding chain and she planned to stonewall our request. Not so easy.

The page from Dr. Brown's office to me that morning must mean the cat was out of the bag. As a new attending, a call to the medical director's office was not a good thing. It was like a summons to the principal's office in junior high. I ran to my office and grabbed a rumpled tie that I kept around for occasions like this. Sometime during this period I began to wear a tie regularly, because I thought it was disrespectful to put a tie on for an administrator and not for a patient. I sat outside Dr. Brown's office and waited for the summons to enter. A young administrative assistant walked out. "Dr. Ansell, Dr. Brown will see you now," she beckoned. I followed her into the office.

Dr. Rowine Brown, the medical director, was a long-term County physician, a fixture from the late 1940s. She was gray-haired, well-coiffed, and pearled. She had the carriage of a high-society matron and was tough as nails. Given the male chauvinist world of medicine in which she trained and practiced, she must have come by her tempered steel disposition honestly. She sat behind a large, uncluttered desk, in a giant and elegantly appointed office on the second floor of the County Hospital building, overlooking Harrison Street and Pasteur Park to the north. The outsized windows with their patina of soot and pigeon droppings, filtered the light and traffic sounds. In the background, the patter of typing from an IBM Selectric in the office next door punctuated the air. Dr. Brown was known to be an unyielding guardian of the status quo. And proud of it. You messed with her at your own peril.

It was clear that the "rules" prevented new programs from ever being created in the ossified County system. We would have to break the rules if we were to succeed. Our residency training served us well in this regard. Many times, over the past four years, I had to break the rules in order to get the right things done for my patients. Our organizing skills, honed over years of medical school and residency, trained us for these moments. Of course there would be obstacles. We also possessed a natural abhorrence for authority, which helped as well. We refused to take no for an answer. We tried the "right channels." They did not work. Now it was time to dredge a new one.

It was an electric period in Chicago. Harold Washington, a progressive black congressman, was in a tight three-way race in the Democratic primary for mayor of the city. There had never been a black mayor in Chicago. I canvassed for his campaign in the Lakeview precinct where I lived, ringing doorbells house by house to solicit votes. I had a four-block area that I worked after hours and on weekends, knocking on doors and talking to voters. By the time Election Day arrived, we were optimistic that he could pull out a win. He was running against two scions of the despised Democratic Machine. Washington's opponents were Richard Daley, the son of the former mayor, and Jane Byrne, the current mayor who ran as a reformer but converted back to a "business as usual" type once elected. Daley made his name as state's attorney, a law and order tough guy. His prosecutors railroaded a number of men to Death Row on the basis of confessions obtained under torture by police commander John Burge. The Death Row convictions obtained by Daley's states attorneys based on these torture-induced confessions were overturned two decades later. But they made a nice story when young Richie Daley ran for mayor. There was evidence that Daley knew about these torture allegations but chose not to investigate them.

The odds were against a black mayor winning in the most racially polarized city in the U.S. But with two white politicians splitting the white vote, Washington could win if he captured the black and Latino vote along with the white liberal lakeshore residents. The day before the budget hearings were held at the County Building, Washington won the primary election by capturing all the black vote, half the Latino vote and a sliver of the white vote. It was a topsy-turvy time. Washington's win buckled the knees of the Democratic Machine and the reverberations of the win were in the air at the budget hearings.

Arthur had organized a number of people to testify on behalf of the nurses for the breast cancer screening program. He and I were going to testify as well and ask the County Commissioners to add funding for the two nurses to the budget. Arthur had worked behind the scenes with the sympathetic County Commissioner who agreed to speak in support of our request at the board hearing, but she did not guarantee any other votes. It was a long shot, a three-pointer from midcourt at the buzzer, but worth the gamble. There were no other options. As far as we knew, positions had never been added to the budget from the floor of the County chambers.

These public hearings had always been at the focal point of political discourse. As house staff, we routinely signed up to express our opinions along with other union and community members and to show support for adequate funding for the County Hospital. It had been less common for attending physicians to speak at these hearings. But our group of attending physicians, especially those of us who had been student and resident activists, were always ready to speak, much to the dismay of the hospital leadership. When Arthur and I signed up to testify, it must have set off alarms downtown, as well as at the hospital.

"Dr Ansell," Dr. Brown asked. She wasted no time on formalities, "Why have you signed up to testify at the Budget hearings?"

I forced a wan smile. When I told her it was to ask for the nurse positions, she scowled.

"Dr. Ansell," she said, in a voice reminiscent of Tallulah Bankhead, "you have bypassed all the regular channels." Her gray eyes, peering from over the tops of the bifocals perched halfway down her aquiline nose, raked me over. She was not happy.

"You will never succeed at County if you do not play by the rules. Do not go down and ask for positions that are not in the budget." It was an awkward moment. I listened politely but did not agree to her demand. The hearings were open to the public. Anyone could testify. My job felt safe, even if my relationships with my superiors did not.

The monumental classical revival style City Hall-County Building took up an entire city block. The west side held the offices of the mayor, city clerk, city treasurer, some city departments, aldermen, and the Chicago City Council. The east side was the Cook County Building. The foyer and great hall were illuminated by a light that exuded an emerald Oz-like glow. The elevators were bright brass. The entrance on Clark Street faced the orange metal Picasso bull that occupied a portion of the Daley Plaza across the street, site of our many demonstrations to keep County Hospital open. The County Board chambers where the hearings were held were located on the fifth floor. On one end of the floor was the Office of the President of the County Board. On the other side was the Office of Mayor of Chicago. This was the belly of the beast of the Chicago Democratic Machine. The County Board chambers were packed. In the front was a raised dais where the County Board President, the Chairman of the Finance Committee and their aides sat. Below was a semi-circular area where the other county commissioners convened in swivel chairs behind dark-stained wooden desks. Behind that area, separated by a railing, was the seating area for the public. It was filled with union representatives, community activists, and reporters. Behind the seats, people were standing. I found a seat and waited for my name to be called. I had prepared a written testimony about the problem of breast cancer and the request for the two nurses to get a breast cancer screening program started. I was not a confident public speaker growing up. Four years earlier, I had gotten stage fright and mangled my words in front of a crowd. But training at County toughened me. Arthur's presence helped as well.

The hearings were being chaired by an old-time County Board political hack, a crony of George Dunne and the Chairman of the Finance Committee of the County Board. He was indicted for mail fraud and would be sentenced the next year to a stint in federal prison. He was one of many in a long tradition of Cook County politicians who, having gorged themselves at the public trough, got caught and were sent to jail. He would eventually be forced to relinquish his County Board seat for a prison jumpsuit. My name was called. The hum of voices in the chambers dimmed as I walked up to the speaker's podium. I had three minutes to make my case. Dr. Brown, a pillar of ice, sat near the podium and telegraphed me the evil eye just as she had done to Dr. Hoffman before me. I stated the case for breast cancer screening for the patients at Cook County Hospital, reading my prepared testimony.

The indicted commissioner was the first to speak after my testimony. "Doc", he asked, in Chicago patois, "didya take dis request, troo da proper channels? You know, we can't consider dis unless it has been troo da channels."

I stared at him in disbelief. Here was a guy about to go to prison for fraud, for violating the trust of his office, for cheating, and he asked me about the proper channels? I bit my tongue to keep myself from laughing at the irony of the situation. Channels? He could teach me a thing or two about channels.

Just then, our supporter on the Board jumped in with the story about her breast cancer survival and threw her support to this program. Others chimed in as well. It touched an emotional chord with the Board. The electricity in the air from the election of Harold Washington had helped us. The vote for the program occurred at a finance committee meeting a few weeks later. I have saved the transcript of that meeting, sent to me by the aide to our supporter. The vote was not even close. At the vote, George Dunne, the County Board president revealed, "I am a cancer survivor, too. I had colorectal cancer. I will support this program." It was a done deal, if President

Dunne said yes; it was in the bank. The budget was published with two new nursing positions for breast cancer screening. The Breast Cancer Screening Program was born.

CHAPTER 15

1984: The Breast Cancer Screening Program

IN 1984, Ms. MC, a 39 year-old African American woman with no health insurance, found a lump in her left breast. Desperate and in fear for her life, she took a bus across Chicago's West Side to the Emergency Room at Cook County Hospital. County Hospital, her hospital. The "best doctors," they'd see her. But she had to wait. The waiting was worst for those with chronic diseases. Those with emergencies were seen first. County was nationally recognized for its Trauma and Burn Services. But those with non-emergency problems went to the end of the line. When you were seen, it was likely a doctor in training or a medical student who made the assessment and prescribed the treatment. There were not enough senior physicians to see all the patients. Sometimes the young doctors made the right call and sometimes not. This was the lot of the uninsured in Chicago.

MC lingered half a day to be seen, on a hard wooden seat in the Emergency Room waiting area. She strained to hear her name called above the din of the waiting room. She thought of leaving. Every day, others like her got up and walked out in disgust. Sick and tired of being sick, and tired. "LWOTs" they are called; Left Without Treatment. A statistic, and not a good one. Some think that those who walk out without being seen must not have needed care. But studies have tracked these people and they have a higher rate of hospitalization and complexity than the general population. MC came to the County Emergency Room because there were no doctor's offices in the neighborhoods to treat her. It might not have been an emergency but she had nowhere else to go.

MC stayed. Her fear kept her planted. "MC!" her name blared over the loudspeaker. It was her time. A young doctor led her into an examination room. A brief history was taken. The doctor examined her breasts. On the left side was a large, hard lump. Likely a cancer, the doctor told her. Go to the breast clinic. They will follow up.

MC later told me of the swirl of thoughts and emotions that filled her. A knot of fear twisted her gut when she heard the dreaded word "cancer." The big "C." A word not uttered in the black community. It meant death. A sucker punch. Her worst fear. It was as if all the neurons in her brain had short circuited. She did not remember much else of the visit, she was so overcome with terror. The dread of losing her breast. How would her husband react? The terror that her young son might grow up without a mother. Like many women facing this moment, she was thinking of those closest to her, not of herself. Later, when she began to work with me as a volunteer in the Breast Cancer Screening Clinic, she taught me that the women were not able to hear a word I said in the moments after I told them that they might have breast cancer. She would see the women after I broke the news and spend time with them bringing them the perspective of a survivor and patient advocate, a woman who had been through it all—biopsy, mastectomy, chemotherapy—and made it to the other side.

But at that moment in the Cook County Emergency Room her future was unclear. She trudged to the Breast Clinic to make an appointment. Her hopes were dashed again. Located on the third floor of Fantus Clinic, the outpatient clinic building attached to County Hospital, the waiting room was a sea of women and men sprawled on benches and leaning against the walls. MC, the pink discharge slip from the Emergency Room clutched in her hand, jostled through the swarm of people gathered near the entrance of the clinic and squeezed herself to the desk of the clerk, where she joined a throng of women who were also trying to get appointments. When her turn came, the clerk took the form from MC's hand, looked it over and checked the paper log for the next appointment for the breast doctor. She wrote the appointment on a white slip and handed it to MC. Three months. MC was staggered by this news. She could not wait three months. The cancer would spread. Panic filled her chest. She gathered herself, leaned over and whispered to the clerk about her condition. She begged for an earlier appointment. The clerk, a County veteran, was not moved. Numbed over the years by the press of patients and their demands, she had heard it all. "Take it or leave it."

MC trudged toward the Fantus exit. Not sure of her plans. On the wall, by the elevator, a ragged notice caught her eye. An act of God. "Attention All Women," it declared. "If you have a problem or concern about your breasts, call the Breast Cancer Detection Program." Days before, we had just started the program and put signs up to notify women. MC found her way to the program that next Friday. I examined her and referred her for treatment. Later, after a mastectomy and chemotherapy, MC became a volunteer.

In 1984, in the weeks before MC first came to County, we started the Breast Cancer Detection program. Arthur was helpful. He taught me how to get the breast cancer screening program started. It was "see one, do one, teach one" all over again, just like residency.

Once a position was listed in the County Budget it was as good as gold. That's how the patronage Machine greased its skids. They slipped a position in the budget under a cost center. People showed up on the payroll. Maybe they came to work and maybe they did not. They were relatives or friends of politicians. Or get-out-the-vote types. It was the story of County. It was hard to know how widespread the patronage extended at County. But occasionally the same rules worked for the good. The two nurse positions were listed in the budget. Under a new cost center. I was in charge by default. Oh boy! I had no idea what I had gotten myself into!

I began to interview nurses for the program and hired two passionate nurses who led the program from its inception until they retired. Jackie Dillard was a nurse who grew up picking cotton in Jim Crow Yazoo City, Mississippi. She came to Chicago as a teenager. Before she came to County, she once confided in me, she had never worked with a white man. She was shy and tentative during the interview and I was not sure if I should hire her. At the end of the interview she looked me in the eye and said, "Dr. Ansell, you won't be disappointed if you hire me." I hired her, and I was not disappointed. Jackie ultimately became the program manager. The other nurse, Marcia Rothenberg, was a former County nurse, a breast cancer survivor who had been active in the civil rights and peace movements. She was about four foot ten inches tall, a peripatetic and outspoken woman topped with a bird's nest of gray wiry hair. Together, the three of us designed the program from scratch.

The nurses commandeered a large examination room and filled it with chairs. Then, twice a day they scoured the waiting room and recruited women to join the class on breast health. There were two commodities in great supply at County: waiting time and our patients' desire to learn. Classes were planned for early morning and afternoon while the women were waiting to see their doctors. Like a Broadway producer, I walked past the classroom where Marcia and Jackie were going to teach, wringing my hands, wondering if the women would show up. I was thrilled. The seats were packed with women. Some stood against the wall. They clutched the educational brochures we had designed. It was a hit.

The room's ventilation system was not designed for crowds this size and it soon shimmered with heat. Day after day the scene was repeated. The women were hungry for health education, not only about breast cancer but also menopause and other subjects. Over 600 women attended classes in the first twenty days. By the end of the first year, Jackie and Marcia had taught, examined and sent thousands of women for screening mammograms. We began to see women with advanced breast cancer who had waited months to get into the breast surgery clinic but whom we now saw within two weeks.

The Breast Cancer Screening Program began to attract attention as it was one of the first in the U.S. The issue of black-white disparities in cancer outcomes was just beginning to gain notice on the national scene. The literature on breast cancer suggested that black women had fatalistic attitudes, lacked knowledge and avoided treatment. While we certainly saw some women who fit that description, we could not help but think our health-care system itself was responsible for keeping a black woman like MC from needed treatment for three months. Those of us who practiced in the underbelly of the U.S. health care system believed it was institutionalized racism and the lack of a universal health care system, not just bad attitudes, that accounted for the poor health outcomes we saw.

Like many things we did at County, there was usually resistance and sometimes conflict when we tried to change the way in which care was delivered. Our superiors viewed us as an ornery, obstinate and argumentative bunch. We were always bucking the status quo, or so it seemed. But we believed that we were providing the care that our patients deserved. The history of County was littered with these patient care innovations—first resisted and then accepted, oftentimes national models of care delivery. The first blood bank in the world, the first trauma unit, preventive medicine programs, care for patients with AIDS and addictions. The Breast Cancer Screening Program was one of these.

Now we found ourselves in a fight to improve the care delivered to all women with breast cancer at the hospital. The surgeons saw me as an interloper. Who was this guy Ansell? In their minds, I had popped up out of nowhere and they were not happy. They were the experts in breast cancer treatment. I was encroaching on their turf. The Breast Surgery Clinic was not very functional. Women could not get in for months. It was a mill. Rather than subject our patients to this, I insisted that a surgeon come to our clinic to see the patients who needed biopsies. Our nurses would do the first evaluation. If they had concerns, I would see them and I would refer only the ones I had questions about to the surgeons. The surgeons relented and began to show up.

Then I crossed a line with the surgeons, one that needed to be crossed, about the treatment of breast cancer. In the early 1980s at

County Hospital, women were still being treated with radical mastectomies. Women were not getting breast-conserving surgery, the state-of-the-art surgical treatment by that time. I was told by a breast surgeon that the County patients would bleed to death if they went home with lumpectomies. He thought our patients were not educated enough to care for their wounds. I grimaced when I heard this. At the very least it was disrespectful of our patients; it was more likely racist. I knew if we were going to be doing breast screening that we needed to be providing best-practice breast surgery at County and I was determined to change their practice. But first I had to get the attention of Dr. G, the head of the cancer treatment program at both the University of Illinois and County. Territorial and political, he was one of the most powerful doctors on the medical staff. He had an international reputation as a cancer surgeon, and a local one for always getting his way. He did not know what to make of me. He had been king of the hill when it came to cancer treatment at the two hospitals. I was a pipsqueak. A nobody. An upstart. Who did I think I was, running a breast screening clinic? And telling his surgeons how to treat patients? The surgeons stonewalled me on issues of breast cancer treatment. Then an opportunity arose. One of our patients had received an unnecessary radical mastectomy despite our prior discussion with the surgeons involved with the case. I sent a letter to my superior and the patient's primary care doctor in which I questioned the patient's clinical care. I copied Dr. G at his office at the University of Illinois. Instead of a reply, I was paged to the office of the Medical Director of the Fantus Clinic.

Dr. Agnes Lattimer was a pediatrician who was recently appointed Medical Director of Fantus Clinic. She was a woman in her sixties with a mahogany, sphinx-like face whose surface betrayed little emotion. Lattimer was the only black woman in her medical school class of 1940 and had held a number of medical leadership positions at County before becoming Medical Director of Fantus. Another tough woman who had to overcome the obstacles of sexism and racism to achieve her success, she was a no-nonsense type and a fierce patient advocate. You did not mess with Agnes.

"Someone told me that you are doing breast biopsies. Is this true?" she asked me.

"Yes," I replied. "I am credentialed to do needle biopsies."

I suspected Dr. G was behind this. This was not about my credentials. It was about the letter. Dr. Lattimer pulled my credentials. They were in order. I had made sure that the breast biopsy privileges had been approved.

Then Dr. G retaliated again. He forbade his surgeons to come to my clinic to see the patients with breast cancer. That's when I realized that my letter had touched a raw nerve. We were now worse off than before. They had not changed their minds on surgical treatment and now the patients were relegated to the chaos of the Breast Clinic. I tried to call Dr. G to resolve things, but he refused my calls. Not one to tolerate stonewalling, I hatched a plan. One Friday afternoon, I called over to the U. of I. to make sure that Dr. G was in his office. He was. And he refused to take my call again. Steamed, I walked the two blocks to his office.

His secretary tried to get me to leave, "Dr. G is not here," she lied.

"That's ok, I'll wait," I replied, and took a seat in the waiting area. And waited.

Hours later, my opportunity arose. I saw him sneak out of his office and walk to the copy room. Like a hound dog on a fox chase, I ran past the secretary and cornered him at the copy machine in a supply room off his office. I stood between Dr. G and the door and refused to leave until he agreed to speak. A short, well-dressed man with thinning black hair, a crisp white shirt and sharply pressed trousers, I felt him withdraw in revulsion at my presence. His jet black eyes averted my gaze. I spoke up. I would have to fast-talk to get myself out of this one.

"Dr. G, I'm Dr. Ansell, I need to talk with you about my letter." By his scowl and furrowed brow, I realized how much I had pissed him off.

"I can't talk with you now. I'm busy." He said as he gathered his papers. He looked as if he was about to dash out. Still no eye contact.

"I am sorry if I offended you," I said and held my ground between the copier and the door. He had to pass through me to get out of the room. Eventually, he looked up at me, his eyes glaring. He lectured me like a schoolmaster on my bad manners, wagging his finger, upset that I sent the letter and copied others on it. He was less upset about the care of the patients than he was angry that others had seen the letter critiquing his surgeons' patient care. After an hour of back and forth, he acquiesced to have his surgeons staff my program again. I learned a lesson. Never deliver bad news by letter or email, even if it is true. But in standing my ground, the surgical treatment of the women improved.

The Breast Cancer Screening Program thrived for many years and expanded to include community outreach and mobile vans before funding cutbacks a few years ago reduced its staffing and reach. Jackie and Marcia have long since retired, but the program we started in 1984 still lives on at County Hospital. The Breast Cancer Screening Program was just one of many preventive medicine programs—smoking cessation and stress reduction programs; HIV prevention programs; and later, drug and alcohol counseling programs—that were developed at County despite the opposition of the hospital leadership. We all believed that our patients deserved more than just a hospital to treat late-stage disease. They deserved the best primary care, including the opportunity for the prevention or early detection of diseases. Like the blood bank and the trauma unit, these programs received national recognition as models of care delivery. If we had not pushed back against the status quo none of these innovations in care delivery would have happened. But sometimes even these efforts were not enough.

In 2006, my colleagues and I discovered that, despite efforts like the Breast Cancer Screening Program, black breast cancer mortality had not budged in Chicago since the early 1980s and the Chicago racial gap in breast cancer mortality was the largest in the U.S. Why?

We postulated that the health-care system in Chicago was designed in such a perverse way that black women were still unable to receive the best outcomes despite all the advances in breast cancer care. As a result, hundreds of black women died from breast cancer each year in Chicago because they did not have the same outcomes as white women. Despite the intent of programs like the Breast Cancer Screening Program, regionally it was as if nothing had changed or improved for black women with regard to this disease. There was more work to be done to eliminate this mortality gap and it required the whole health-care system to change, not just one program at the County Hospital. A quarter of a century after Ms. MC first sought care for her breast cancer at our program at County, black women with breast cancer in Chicago still could not expect to have the outcomes that white women have. Martin Luther King Jr. once said, "Of all the forms of inequality, injustice in health is the most shocking and most inhumane." Despite our efforts to achieve equity in breast cancer diagnosis and treatment, we have fallen short in overcoming this injustice.

CHAPTER 16

1985: I'm Sticking to the Union

TWENTY ATTENDING PHYSICIANS sat around tables in the medical staff meeting room on the first floor of the Administration Building. On the far wall, a row of windows overlooked Ogden Avenue where it crossed Damen. Cars whizzed by in the distance. We debated the next steps. We were under siege. Again. A familiar feeling. An attending physician, AB, in the Department of Neurology had developed AIDS. The hospital Medical Director discovered this and decreed that he could have no patient contact. It was an arbitrary and ignorant response to the AIDS epidemic that was sweeping across Chicago. This was a civil rights issue, a call to arms to defend our colleague and our rights.

My friends in the Division of General Medicine had been at the forefront of treating the AIDS epidemic. Two physicians, Ron Sable and Renslow Sherer, started the first outpatient clinic for AIDS patients at County. Mardge Cohen began a clinic for women and children with HIV/AIDS. It was the first in Chicago and one of the first in the U.S. This was the early days of the epidemic and there was no known treatment. What was known was that person-to-person transfer of the virus that causes AIDS could only occur through the exchange of bodily fluids. There was no biological basis for denying this doctor his livelihood.

The County Hospital reeled under the impact this new disease had on patients and staff. Our patients developed unusual and deadly infections we had rarely seen: parasitic pneumonias, brain infections and tuberculosis. They were among the sickest patients in the hospital—young, wasted and cachectic with ribs and joints protruding. Their eyes were sunken like Auschwitz survivors. Our nursing and support staff were terrified of AIDS. Some shunned the patients, not wanting to enter their rooms for fear of contracting the disease. The patients felt isolated, abandoned and demeaned. They were treated like modern-day lepers. The indignity of the conditions of inpatient units added to the despair and loneliness that accompanied the disease. Our physicians worked to educate the staff about AIDS and even created a separate unit to treat AIDS patients. It was not easy. Statewide there were efforts by conservative groups to limit the civil rights of people with AIDS: mandatory tracing of sexual contacts, and screening for HIV without consent. Renslow, Ron and Mardge were at the leading edge of this civil rights debate. They feared that the outing of patients with AIDS would lead to loss of insurance and jobs. They worked with state legislators to write statutes that protected patients against undue prying from government and employers.

It was in this context that limiting the attending physician's privileges and the public outing of him and his disease was so abhorrent. Dr. AB was one of the most respected attending physicians on the medical staff, a great clinician and teacher. Nothing about his clinical work could put patients at risk. None of our physicians, experts in the diagnosis and management of AIDS, were consulted before his suspension. This was the County Hospital and this arbitrary decree to limit his ability to work had been made out of ignorance, the same type of ignorance and fear that affected our staff. The political establishment weighed in on the side of injustice when the County Board President, George Dunne, publicly supported the Medical Director. The medical staff mobilized to oppose the limitations to Dr. AB's practice. We held meetings, demonstrations and ultimately filed a lawsuit. The courts forced County to back off.

In this atmosphere of polarization and administrative fiat, a few of us gathered and decided to try to form a union of attending physicians. In the wake of the attempted suspension of our colleague with AIDS, we did not see a way to guarantee the rights of attending physicians without a labor contract. Peter Orris and I took the lead. With a nasal Upper-West-Side New York accent, thinning gray hair and a paunch, Peter was a veteran of the civil rights and antiwar movement and a physician in the occupational medicine division. He had been a leader in the House Staff strike as a first-year resident, in 1975. We decided to convene a small group of physicians and psychologists to gauge interest in a union. The recent decree against our colleague was still fresh in our minds when we met. Many of the attending physicians appointed in the past five or six years had been members of the House Staff Association, the resident union, and realized the benefits that derived from unionization. The transition from resident to attending meant that we lost some of the advantages we had with the House Staff union.

The full-time attending physician at County Hospital was a recent occurrence. Prior to the 1970s there were few full-time attendings at County. Most were on the staffs of other hospitals and worked part-time teaching at County. Even when I became an attending, in 1983, many of the senior physicians on staff practiced elsewhere. But there were a growing number of attending physicians like me, whose only employment was at County. We viewed our practices at County as long-term careers and wanted the greater sense of security that a union might bring.

The move to unionize attending physicians in the U.S. was a relatively new phenomenon and the major unions were looking to garner some wins among employed physicians. The State of Illinois had recently passed a law that set down the conditions that made it possible for public employees to organize unions. A State Labor Board was created to adjudicate these efforts. Recently, the public defenders, lawyers working for the County, had successfully unionized, making ripe the conditions for an attending physician union drive at County.

We had two options. We could try to organize ourselves as an independent union—an attending version of the unaffiliated House

Staff Association, or we could affiliate with a national union that would provide the muscle, money and staff to organize us. There was a vociferous debate on this subject. On the one hand, there was some feeling that attending physicians might be uncomfortable being in the same union as the clerical staff and others at the hospital. In many ways this elitism was at the heart of the debate around the value of unions for attending physicians. These doctors, most of whom made close to six-figure salaries, did not fit the usual mold of a working-class labor union. And in a hospital, their interests had more often than not been aligned with management than with front-line workers. This was not true at County Hospital where most physicians were battling an unresponsive, disengaged and politicized management. And other professionals such as lawyers and college professors had unions.

We invited two established unions to present their credentials to us. After this selection we would organize the rest of the doctors with the financial and organizational clout of a major union. Organizing a union is straightforward. We needed to get a majority of the attending physicians to sign cards. These cards would be presented to the hospital administration along with a petition to hold a secret ballot election among all the attending physicians. If the majority of those who turned out voted yes, we would win. Not so easy. We knew that the County Board would challenge our unionization attempt by claiming we were supervisors. If we were to succeed, the State Labor Board had to agree with our petition for a union. But that was a long way off. This was the first battle.

If the issue were to get to the Labor Board, we needed to win two of the three votes. One was a labor-appointed member. We should have that vote. The second was appointed by the Chicago Mayor, Harold Washington, the anti-Machine Democrat. Not sure about this one but we thought we should be able to get it as well. The third vote was controlled by the Governor of Illinois, a Republican, who would most certainly vote against us. It was a long road ahead but we could taste the victory.

The first union we considered was the American Federation of State, County and Municipal Employees (AFSCME), one of the largest unions in the country. They represented public employees all around the nation. AFSCME had the advantage of being a major union in the county with a large Chicago presence including the County Hospital. A couple of AFSCME union officials, dressed in two-piece suits came to talk with us. Many of us mistrusted the coziness between the Chicago unions and the corrupt Democratic political Machine that controlled the County Board. They turned me off with their talk of their local connections. But from a pragmatic perspective, they had clout. And in Chicago, clout mattered.

The second union was 1199, a progressive health-care union out of New York City. It represented only people who worked in health care and had some unionized doctors. 1199 had no Chicago ties. This had some advantages. A number of attending physicians we needed to convince would not sign a card to join a union that was the same union that represented the ward clerks. An outfit from the outside had the advantage of not having ties to the dreaded Democratic Machine. Since 1199 had no other plans to organize in Chicago, they could represent our interests without having to be concerned about competing bargaining units. We liked their style. The national President, Henry Nicholas, and his vice president for organizing, flew to Chicago to woo us, an impressive display of their interest.

The decision was close. There were strong voices on both sides. But 1199 carried the day. It was an appeal to the heart that did it. Michael Cohen, a goateed, slightly built pediatrician, his thin brown hair tied into a neat pony tail, stood up in front of us. He was a precise speaker and he addressed the gathering of physicians from the varied departments. He took us back almost two decades. It was 1966, he was a high school student in New York attending his first march against the Vietnam War. All eyes were on him as he described that march in New York City in the early spring. A warm and sunny day. Most unions would not join the demonstration because at that time they supported the government and the war effort. But one did:

1199. 1199 was the first labor union in the U.S. to oppose the war in Vietnam. We listened as Michael described the experience of being one of fifty thousand people marching down 34th Street. And there, near the front of the march, were a multi-racial group of hundreds of hospital workers, holding 1199 banners, yelling "End the War" as they marched past Gimbels and Macy's. Many physicians in the room had come of age in the anti-war movement. The emotional connection between 1199, the anti-war movement and our unionization attempt moved the undecided. I cast my vote for 1199 and they won. Much to the chagrin of the AFSCME leadership who had done so much to court us, local clout lost. It was a decision that we would second-guess many times.

Peter Orris and I were experienced organizers. And we were organizing against a corrupt and politicized administration. You could not make up a better opponent. A county-appointed hack was running the hospital. By the time of the selection of 1199 we had identified and organized physician and psychologist representatives from all the major departments and had begun to meet frequently. There were a few hundred attending physicians at County. We began to set up small group meetings of physicians to discuss the benefits of a union and listened to the concerns.

1199 sent two of their best organizers from New York to Chicago for the campaign. Alice Bush, the lead organizer, was adored by the attending physicians. Alice was a plain-speaking, matter-of-fact, no-nonsense type of person. With short brown hair, piercing brown eyes, and pencil-thin lips, she had a wry sense of humor, perfect for County. With Alice's help, we collected signatures from physicians in the fall of 1984. We were able to sign up about sixty percent of the attending physicians, despite the counter-efforts of the hospital leadership to dissuade physicians from joining. But the fun was just beginning.

In April 1985, a small group of us delivered the signed cards to the hospital administration with a request that the County authorize an election. We had been organizing the campaign for over a year. We were optimistic that we would have a union within a short period.

Now the real fight began in front of the Labor Board. The County's lawyers fought our request for a union, tooth and nail. They forced us to hold extensive hearings over many months to determine the scope, breadth and legal legitimacy of the union. Physicians with many titles and job descriptions were brought in front of the labor board to testify to their job duties. The County claimed that the attending physicians were supervisors because they supervised residents and thus were ineligible under the law to form a union. We counter-argued that we had no hiring or firing control over residents so we were not supervisors in the true sense of the word. We were teachers and direct patient caregivers and thus eligible for unionization.

The hearings dragged on for a year. Finally, in the summer of 1987 the hearing officer from the Labor Board made his ruling in our favor. Attending physicians at County Hospital were not supervisors and therefore had the right to unionize. We were jubilant. We had won. But joy turned to jitters when the County appealed the decision to the full Labor Board. As far as we knew, the full Labor Board never overturned a hearing officer's decision. Until now. When the decision of the Labor Board was released, we were shocked. We should have seen this coming.

The Governor's representative on the Board voted against us, as we had expected. The Mayor's representative voted for us. One for, one against. To our shock, the labor vote on the Labor Board voted against us. We were betrayed by organized labor. Little did we know then, but the effort would be set back for years. Another attempt to unionize failed in 1995. It would be twenty-three years before an attending physician union at County Hospital was approved.

Six years later, in 1993, I discovered who was behind the no vote from organized labor. Harry Kirschenbaum was the Director of the Service Employees International Union (SEIU) in Chicago. We were talking on the phone about another matter. SEIU had its roots in Chicago and had grown since the 1920s into a large national union. SEIU represented the clerks at Cook County Hospital. Harry was a fist-banging, cigar-chomping, pinky-ring-wearing, Chicago union boss. A battle-scarred veteran of countless labor wars. Ruthless and vengeful, he had been a leader on the Chicago labor scene for over fifty years. I asked him if he knew why organized labor blocked our unionization attempt. I stirred a hornet's nest of emotion with my inquiry.

"You're goddamn right I know. I blocked the vote," he said, as if still stung by the memory.

I listened, shocked. "Why did you block the vote?" I asked.

"You had no business bringing 1199 into Chicago. They were outsiders. They didn't belong. That's why," he said.

Our choice of 1199 to represent us turned out to have doomed this first unionization attempt. Harry was furious that 1199 would dare to come into Chicago, into his hospital, and organize. Harry had clout. And he used it. To screw us. The Labor vote on the state Labor Board was held by a Harry Kirshenbaum crony. Harry muscled him to vote against us. A union-organizing campaign stymied by organized labor. We were taken to the woodshed. Only in Chicago.

One good outcome from this organizing effort was a report on the future of the Cook County Health System that was written by a coalition of unions including the attending physicians. At this time there was no consensus on the future of the hospital. Certainly there was no vision for what the County Health System could be. As far as we knew, in the past 150 years there had never been a strategic plan for the County Health System. So we wrote one, "A Proposal for a Public Health System for Cook County." The proposal was far-reaching. Not just a plan for a replacement hospital on the West Side, but a system of care that was regional, comprehensive and emphasized primary and preventive care as well as hospital services. It proposed a new County Hospital to be built on the West Side campus, a smaller South Side hospital, and a network of community clinics, all linked with community health centers and the health clinics run by the City of Chicago into one system of care. It emphasized community-based primary care. It presaged what the Cook County Health System would approach at its zenith seventeen years later, but in 1986 was only a dream. My picture was on the front of the proposal. It received some press coverage on its release and then quickly was relegated to some back shelf to collect dust.

In the end, I had mixed feelings about the attending union. As attending physicians, we still had a lot of privilege in the County system, even without union protections. Besides, the union alone would not address the larger issues of underfunding and political interference that plagued the hospital. A union offered a way to have a more collective voice against an arbitrary administration, but I was not sure if it would lead to meaningful improvement at the hospital. In subsequent organizing campaigns, I did not play as active a role. By the late 1980s I had moved on to the most challenging and disturbing job of my career: running the sprawling walk-in clinic at County.

CHAPTER 17

1989–1992:
Designed to Fail

"CAN YOU SIGN OFF a chart for me?" the nurse practitioner asked.

"Sure, what do you have?" I replied.

I was on duty in the Ambulatory Screening Clinic, County's walk-in clinic. I sat on a rolling stool in the work area, encircled by a group of nurses, charts in hand, who waited to swoop in at the next opening for me to sign off on their cases. The overhead page blared every thirty seconds, an electronic stress test that throttled my heart rate with each tinny blast.

An outbreak of measles had been reported in the U.S. I read the "Morbidity and Mortality Weekly Reports," a publication of the Centers for Disease Control as if it were a Bible. They reported epidemics. If a disease spread anywhere in the world, it would find its way to this Chicago walk-in-clinic. Malaria. Tuberculosis. AIDS. Domestic violence. We had seen it all. It was just a matter of time before we would see a case of measles. I was a teenager during the last outbreak in the 1960s. No one else in my group had seen a case either. Measles is a disease that is highly contagious and is spread by the coughing of infected droplets. Patients with measles present with cough, red eyes, runny nose and a rash on the face, body and inside the mouth. In the 1950s and 1960s children got it, now it was infecting young adults. It could be misdiagnosed as bronchitis or just a bad cold. I found an old-time infectious diseases doctor and asked him for some photos of patients splattered with the characteristic splotchy measles rash. I stuck them on the bulletin boards like "FBI Most Wanted" posters at the post office.

Some of the nurses who worked in the clinic were excellent. Other nurse practitioners who worked in the clinic were jaded and cynical. Some were mean to patients. Hardened and devoid of empathy, this one particular nurse who wanted me to sign the chart was not a strong clinician. She had bleached blond hair, lacquered with spray into a cotton-candy beehive. Her baby-blue eyes, the color of the Caribbean, had a vacant and emotionless stare. None of the docs trusted her. She had been suspected in the past of making up her patient notes. I had to discipline her on more than one occasion because of patient complaints. She was not too fond of me and avoided me like a contagion. So when she presented this case to me, I was primed to be suspicious.

"I have a guy with a *Bactrim* rash. You don't need to see him." She shoved the chart in front of my face for me to sign. Not so fast.

"Tell me more," I said. The nurse hurled me an azure-blue evil-eye and then rattled off the case.

"He's a 23-year-old who was here last week for bronchitis and was treated with *Bactrim*. Now he's back with a rash. Likely from *Bactrim*. I stopped the med and started him on *Benadryl.*" She shoved the chart back in front of me, again.

Hmm. *Bactrim* was the brand name for a sulfa antibiotic. It could cause a rash. But a young man with bronchitis sick enough to get antibiotics and a new rash sounded suspicious. This could be measles. I insisted on seeing the patient despite the nurse's protestations. I pushed open the examination room door. A young guy, sick as a dog, sat on the examination table breathing rapidly. His eyes were vampire red and rheumy. He coughed. A high-pitched Jack Russell terrier bark. I could visualize a million measles droplets blasting through our air vents. I handed him a mask to wear. A faint polka dot rash traversed his face and his abdomen. His chest crackled with every breath. Pneumonia. We admitted him to the hospital. My first case of measles.

I was the Director of the Ambulatory Screening Clinic, the walk-in clinic at County Hospital. The Breast Cancer Screening Program had taken off and I was ready to take on another challenge. My friends thought I was nuts to take this on. A fair diagnosis, the problems of the walk-in clinic were thought to be intractable. They were right. The last guy to run it departed, burned-out and depressed. In 1989, I had been at County for eleven years. I was thirty-seven years old. The first strands of gray were peeking through my curly hair. Running the walk-in-clinic placed me at the front lines of one of the most troublesome aspects of the medical care system in the United States: the large numbers of people without primary-care physicians. This clinic provided a front-row seat to the palpable unfairness of health care in America. I threw myself into it.

The clinic treated walk-in patients from seven in the morning until eleven at night. They washed up on the banks of County Hospital like flotsam. The broken and battered. Someone they knew took an interest in their health and said, "Go to County." Or they realized on their own that whatever had been ailing them had reached a point of no return. They came when they could wait no more. Sometimes it was too late. If you needed care in Chicago and you had no insurance, the screening clinic at County would see you for free. You got on a bus, headed for the Loop, and transferred to the Harrison Street bus, which emptied its wounded passengers in front of the clinic door. You walked in, took a number, waited, waited some more, and then some. An eight-hour wait for a fifteen-minute audience with a doctor or nurse was par for the course.

A clinic that began as an afterthought in the early 1970s as more and more people began to walk-in at the Cook County Emergency Room for routine medical care had mushroomed—thanks to the growing ranks of the uninsured. Doctors were added and the hours were extended. Over eighty thousand patients came each year, making it one of the largest clinics in the country. The growth in volume was not a consequence of our stellar customer service. It was a reflection of the deterioration of the health-care safety net in Chicago. Doctor's offices which once peppered the neighborhoods had shuttered, leaving no place for people to receive routine care. Vast swaths of the city from Fullerton Avenue on the North Side to the far South suburbs, twenty miles away, had been designated by the Federal Government as physician-shortage areas. Patients without insurance were rebuffed at other hospitals and clinics and were told to go to Cook County Hospital. Those in ambulances were shipped to the Emergency Room. Those who could walk staggered into the screening clinic. The waiting line for the clinic began at five or six in the morning and trailed down the corridor between Fantus and the hospital. It looked like a soup kitchen line from a Depression-era photo.

A large waiting area, 100 feet long, fronted the clinic, with row upon row of brown wooden seats, many in disrepair. The seats, brand new in 1983, were now breaking off their metal frames like crumbled teeth in a meth addict's mouth. Here an arm rest, there a seat. Bayonets of jagged metal chair frame jutted out, and nurses taped these gaps between seats with white medical adhesive tape on which was written the words, "Don't Sit." It looked like a *CSI* crime scene. In 1992, I got one of the building engineers to trash our broken seats and replace them with the sturdy laminated plywood benches that were used for patient seating during the early days of my residency. These solid church pews were indestructible and had withstood the test of time for twenty-five years or so in Fantus Clinic, but were now being replaced. I reclaimed them from the junk pile. Between the loudspeaker din and the voices of doctors and nurses calling patients, it was hard to hear. Some detractors called this place the "Screaming" Clinic because of its noise level and periodic eruptions from angry customers.

The inside of the clinic was remarkable for its stark antiseptic white appearance. A doctor colleague, who as a medical student had been tortured in the 1970s by the military junta in Argentina, observed that the white paint and glare from the fluorescent lights reminded her of the room in which she was tortured. In response, I had a magenta stripe painted around the inside wall of the clinic.

These were the front lines of everything that was wrong with health care in America. It was a war. And we were losing. If you wanted to make a case for a fair health-care system in the U.S., you needed to spend a day in the Ambulatory Screening Clinic. Walk-in care could be tricky. There was not much time to spend with patients; many others were waiting and we had to move quickly. Most patients had no regular medical care. Over half the patients had untreated hypertension. The patient came in with a rash or a cold. The nurse checked the blood pressure. It was sky high. We did a study. Forty percent of the high blood pressure we detected in men was new. They never knew it. Twenty percent in women was new. These patients needed primary care doctors, not a walk-in clinic. But they were uninsured. We had few places to send them. The General Medicine Clinic had a waiting list of 10,000 patients. That was not a realistic option.

Life expectancy for black males in Chicago was less than sixty-five years, lower than men in Bangladesh. These men died before they collected Social Security or Medicare. The patients, mostly black, who arrived at the walk-in-clinic for medical attention had high rates of undetected chronic diseases—uncontrolled hypertension, diabetes and late stage cancers. They were destined to become the death statistics that epidemiologists collect. As we waded through the endless sea of patients day after day we knew this way of delivering care contributed to early mortality in Chicago. But the next patient was waiting. Who had time to fix it?

There were other epidemics. A patient presented with a sore throat. We could not figure out the cause. We read through all the possible etiologies in the red, dog-eared *Harrison's Textbook of Medicine* we kept in the clinic. There near the bottom of the list of differential diagnoses was syphilis. An ancient, sexually transmitted disease. Bingo! Her syphilis test was positive. We treated her with penicillin and she improved. Little did we know that her case was the leading edge of an epidemic. Each week hundreds of people came to the walk-in clinic with symptoms of sexually transmitted diseases. By the time they were seen and treated, they did not want to wait around to be tested for syphilis and HIV. The "Morbidity and Mortality Weekly Reports" from the Centers for Disease Control detailed a spiking epidemic of new syphilis cases in the U.S. Chicago was at the epicenter of the epidemic. Armed with this information, we sent all the patients who presented with symptoms of sexually transmitted diseases to get their blood tested for syphilis before they were seen. A nurse tracked all the results. Soon our clinic was diagnosing about fifteen percent of the new syphilis cases in all of Cook County, more cases than many states reported. The numbers of new patients with AIDS rose as well. Almost five percent of our patients with syphilis were co-infected with HIV.

One patient haunts me from that time. I walked into the examination room. A young woman, maybe thirty-four or thirty-five. She had a few kids. No insurance. At first blush the symptom seemed minor. But it veiled a more ominous diagnosis.

"What's wrong?" I asked.

"I keep getting urinary tract infections, I think I have another one."

She looked healthy. But she was correct. I checked the computer and she had been to the clinic three or four times with an infection. Each time she had been treated with the correct antibiotics.

"Have you had any other infections?" I inquired.

"No," she replied. "Just the urinary infections."

I checked her urine and she had another infection. Frequent bacterial infections could represent an immune system abnormality. I sent her for an HIV test. It was positive. She had AIDS. We diagnosed many new cases of AIDS in that clinic.

We tried to get as many patients as we could into primary care at County or in the community. But the onslaught of new patients was greater than our efforts could accommodate. Patients like the one with newly-diagnosed AIDS should have had a regular doctor, but she had to return multiple times to the walk-in clinic before we diagnosed her. Each time she was seen by a different doctor. It was not how primary care should work. She was lucky not to fall through the cracks of this crazy system.

As soon as one patient was successfully referred out, there was another to take his or her place. It took extraordinary personal effort to make sure that the patients received the specialty care they needed. If they were allowed to go through the usual processes of referral, they would not be seen on time. So we jumped on the phone, cajoled and finagled to get our patients in. It was a screwed-up system that was dependent on individual doctor intervention. Folks suffered as a result of delays.

As I eyed the long line of patients queing up early each morning to be seen in the walk-in clinic, my stomach gnawed and churned. How would I manage the chaos and unpredictability of the clinic today? Did we have enough staff to handle the load? Some of my anxiety came from my realization that if there were twenty of me, we still could not fix this. At County we were eyewitnesses to the injustice of an apartheid health-care system in Chicago—separate and unequal. We witnessed the brutality that poverty, lack of insurance and racism wrought on patient's bodies and lives. We had come to County because we thought we could fix it. If enough of us came—we could fix it. If we believed enough—we could fix it. If we rallied and protested enough—we could fix it. But I had met my match. The walk-in clinic was unfixable. It was difficult for me to admit failure. The clinic was a symptom of a diseased and failing health-care system. Even I could not fix that.

The one bright light was the change in the administration of the County Health System which occurred during this period. The early 1990s were a Renaissance of sorts at County. George Dunne, the long-time County Board President and Democratic Machine politician, retired and was replaced by Richard Phelan, a reformer. Phelan ran a campaign that had two major promises. Fire the incompetent hack that ran the hospital, and fund the Breast Cancer Screening Program I helped start. His most brilliant move was to bring Ms.

Ruth Rothstein, an experienced hospital administrator, to manage Cook County Hospital. The first competent hospital director we had ever seen. She brought a new era of professional management and much-needed leadership to the health system. Her team stabilized the finances and regulatory threats to the hospital. For the first time, they developed a vision for the future of the County Health System and reached out to us. Now, our efforts at patient care improvements were embraced not repelled.

Rothstein's team created a strategic plan that envisioned an expanded ambulatory care network around the county and a replacement hospital. This plan incorporated many of the ideas we had put forth in the union coalition plan seven years prior. Many of us had long espoused the need for more primary care options for our patients. By the mid 1990s there was a network of sixteen community-based-primary care clinics in the County System. But the demands for primary care outstripped even this new capacity. In the walk-in clinic we expanded contacts with private community-based health centers which would accept discharged patients from the Ambulatory Screening Clinic in exchange for pharmaceuticals and specialty referrals. We set up a system to deliver County pharmaceuticals on a monthly basis to these patients at these community health centers. We also worked with the subspecialists at County to develop criteria for subspecialty referrals from the community to County and to get the test results back to the community providers. It was one of the earliest attempts to create an integrated health-care delivery system for the poor and uninsured in Chicago.

But the flow of patients to the Ambulatory Screening Clinic continued unabated despite the expansion of community-based primary care. The demand for services outstripped our ability to build new capacity as the legions of uninsured grew. We were hopeful that these types of system-building efforts would in time help rationalize the public health system. But there was neither the funding nor the infrastructure to keep up with the skyrocketing demands for the services. But all this system building did not change the fundamental flaw at the core of this health-care delivery system for the uninsured. Dr. Don Berwick, the guru of quality health care improvement in the U.S., currently running the Medicare program for the Obama administration, postulated that "every system is designed to give the results you actually get." Was the County Hospital failing our patients by design? We always thought that given the opportunity, the County Health System could be as good as any in the private sector. Once we got patients in, we knew they would get great care, some of the best in Chicago, but was this adequate if our own systems delayed them or could not accommodate all their needs? What did our great care mean, if delays led to worse outcomes, if we could not manage the growing expectations and demands for our care?

I had never considered that our best efforts, our passions and beliefs about fairness in health would come up short. The first rumblings of doubt began to churn in my gut during those years that I ran the Ambulatory Screening Clinic. The tide of the uninsured was greater than any of our solutions to manage it. "Separate but Equal" was a failed national policy for education, transportation and the military. Why should it work for health care? Unlike those other sectors, the outcome of inequality in health care was disability and death. My tension level rose each day as the next swarm of people filled the seats at the Ambulatory Screening Clinic. There was a reason why so many County doctors thought like me, that only a single-payer health care system would solve this problem. We had seen first-hand the damage done by the current system. But for now, there were patients to be seen.

Twenty years later, I returned to the Ambulatory Screening Clinic for a tour. At 6:30 a.m. every day, the line for the walk-in-clinic snaked from the Fantus entrance to Harrison Street. As I walked into the waiting room of the screening clinic I felt goose bumps on the back of my neck. It was as if I had never left. Nothing had changed. If anything, things had gotten worse. The clinic had been expanded. The visits rose to above 100,000 annually in 2006. The waiting room was crammed and tense, just like before. My purloined benches—still there and stuffed with patients. The magenta stripe around the top of the clinic? Still there as well. Someone had repainted it with religious regularity since 1990. I walked into an examination room and saw my reflection in the mirror over the sink. Age lines that traversed my forehead and crow's-feet around my eyes gave credence to the fact that two decades had passed since I ran this place. In the clinic though, it appeared that time had stood still.

CHAPTER 18

I Felt Like a Human Being

"FOR THE FIRST TIME in my life I felt like a human being," she said, as if by revealing this she realized that perhaps she deserved to be treated this way all along.

Mrs. T, now eighty-two years old, had coffee brown skin freckled with age spots. She looked younger than her age with eyes that crinkled and smiled when she spoke, yet at the same time she displayed a wariness that suggested a pain-filled past. A dab of pink lipstick on her lips, just enough to give some color, her hair was coiffed and relaxed, and pulled back into a bun. She was wearing a white button-down blouse and a pressed pair of slacks. Her demeanor was reserved. Controlled. A quiet person. You would never notice her in a crowd. She was not one to volunteer too much. She lived alone now, her husband had passed many years ago and her daughter was her closest family member. We were talking about County Hospital from the patients' perspective. I asked Mrs. T and three other patients to describe their experiences as patients at County over the years.

Mrs. T had been coming to see me since the earliest days of my residency, slipping in and out of my examination room with hardly a ripple. I did not know her very well. Not like some of my other patients whose medical problems and life dramas had become intertwined with my life story. Mrs. T had very few medical problems and in all my time at County, she was never hospitalized. Because she divulged so little about herself and never complained, her past was veiled. When I asked Mrs. T questions about her life she bared herself in small snippets as if the story of her life was not consequential enough to deserve recitation. She deflected attention. Over the years I learned that she loved to travel. Her daughter had married an IBM executive who was sent by that corporation to various international capitals. When Mrs. T retired from her job as a housekeeper in 1990, she began globetrotting, a little old lady from Chicago who until this time had not wandered far from home. Now she had been everywhere—Africa, Asia, Europe—places that were a long way from her birthplace in Alabama. A small town at the end of a dusty road. Dead end. No work. No possibilities. The oppression of Jim Crow and Southern race laws. I remember when she told me of the pride she felt the first time she went to Africa, the birthplace of her ancestors.

She married young. Her husband was a go-getter.

"Let's go to Chicago," he said. "Good jobs. A better life."

So they came in 1950. Rode the Illinois Central and walked out of Union Station into a bustle of multicolored humanity that churned about the Chicago Loop in a frenzy of commercial activity. So different from small-town life in Alabama. To live in Bronzeville, a whole black city unto itself, south of Chicago's Loop. When it came to hospital choices in 1950, there was only one—Cook County Hospital.

"We didn't know no better," she told me. "It was what was expected. We didn't have no insurance or money or nothing so when we needed something we came to County. That's where they told us to go."

She described giving birth in the infamous "Labor Line," the obstetrics floor at County. Sixty years later, as she sat in my office, her eyes welled as she recounted the indignity. She was twenty-two. Her husband had to drop her off on the first floor. No men were allowed in the Labor Line. She was frightened. It was a place that defied description—a cavernous open ward on the fifth floor off the main hallway. She stood outside in the hallway for hours having contractions while she waited for a stretcher to open up in the labor room. Doubled over with contractions she was finally led into the room. North facing windows filtered the light from outside which illuminated, but did not brighten, the atmosphere in the room. The room was wall-to-wall gurneys. Twenty to thirty women, sometimes more. No privacy. Sweat-drenched women, in various stages of labor, screamed in pain. No medications. The screams of one woman triggered a tidal wave of shrieks from other young women on the other gurneys, as the waves of contractions intensified. Nurses and students checked the progress of the women. There were not enough nurses to minister to the patients. Simple amenities like food, washcloths or towels were unavailable. Many of those laboring were children, fourteen or fifteen years old. Others, like Mrs. T, were older but just as terrified. The women roiled and writhed as the contractions grabbed faster and harder. When the time came and a woman began to push her baby out, the nurse grabbed the gurney and pushed it to the delivery room where the woman, beads of perspiration and a wide-eyed look of terror on her face, propelled her baby out in a final blood-curdling screech.

"We were treated like we was animals, like dogs or cows. Not people. You had your baby and they threw the baby at you like a slab of meat. We did not think to question it. We just had to accept it. We came from the South and we did not ask questions. You were never supposed to question a white man so we just accepted this. We didn't know no better."

The Labor Line opened in 1916 when old Cook County first opened and closed in 2002 when the new hospital opened. The rest of the County experience was like this for her as well. It was not just the long lines and the waits. It was the lack of dignity and respect. She appreciated me as her doctor, but there were others who "treated us like a slab of meat," she reiterated. She diverged and described her experiences with doctors in the south.

"Down South, the doctors would wait on you, but if a white woman came in they'd have to go serve her first. Even if there were black women before her. They'd drop you and run. They'd leave you on the table with your legs raised up, until they was through with the white woman. We never questioned it because that's the way it was. When we got to County, we never expected it to be any different."

It did not even cross her mind to question the treatment, though she was humiliated by it. When I asked her how it made her feel, she spoke of her husband, not of herself.

"He had a good job. He was the first black foreman for the Peoples Gas Company in Chicago. But they wouldn't serve him lunch at the diner on 22nd Street. The men who worked for him would eat at the diner and then bring him food while he sat in the truck and waited."

I did not know why she relayed the story of her husband. Maybe it was to let me know that the experience she had at County was not so unusual. The fact that Chicago was very much like the South was confirmed not just by her experience but by her husband's as well. In those days you just had to bear it.

I asked her what it was like for her when she left County in 1995 to follow me to my new clinic, forty-five years after she first came to County for care. She leaned over as if to tell me a secret.

"For the first time in my life, I felt like a human being," she said in a soft voice.

Ms. NW had a different take on County. She came to Chicago as a young child and grew up on Chicago's West side. She did not have the experience of the South to influence her experiences at County. Her first visit to County was in the 1960s. She was in her seventies now, a decade younger than Mrs. T. Her hair was a gray steel wool frizzle, her face a sallow yellow. Worry lines crisscrossed her mouth and eyes. She had many medical problems through the years and had followed me to the three hospitals where I have practiced. Once I asked her about the differences between the three. She ranked them like Zagats.

"Pres—the nurses are real good. Mount Sinai—the best food. Mmm. Mmm. You sat there with your knife and fork in your hands waiting for them to bring it. County," she paused, "ya gotta wait. The service was poor." She spoke of the Emergency Department and what it was like to be a patient there.

"In them days everybody without insurance had to travel to the County. You could be so sick," she groused, "you sit there all day. All day!" she said and drawled out the word day for emphasis. "Until you got better and got up to go home. I did that. Waited and waited so long that I just got better and left." Sometimes the wait was too long. She relayed a story about a friend.

"A lady I knew back then. She was in her twenties. She went to the County because she had pain in her side. She was bent over in pain it was so bad. She lay on that cart all day and all night until her appendix burst. When they got to her she had died. It was kinda bad."

She spoke of how in 1988 she had fallen off a ladder while painting her apartment and broken her shoulder. A neighbor called 911.

"You'd ask the ambulance to take you to another closer hospital and they'd always take you to the County." She speculated that this was because the ambulances worked for County. (They did not—they were part of the city Fire Department.) She spoke of lying on a stretcher in pain in the ER all day and night while she waited to be seen.

"You would call someone and no one come and see you. You on this bed. In pain. Hurtin' because you were there so long. I lay there for more than eight hours. Houngry! Ain't getting nuthin ta eat! No crackers. No water. No bathroom. All day lonnng!" she said.

Finally, in the middle of the night they admitted her and put a cast on her shoulder. She told a similar story of delays in the County ER when she broke her wrist in 2008.

She liked the doctors at County and thought that once she got treated that she received good care. But it was the delays, the lack of basic nursing care and the indignity and the humiliation that bothered her. She spoke of what it was like to be a patient on Ward 35—the admitting ward. That was where I met her in 1978.

"It was so bad, Ward 35. Women right next to mens. They would try to cover you up. But there was no privacy. It was humiliating. They were taking information from you. No privacy at all. You could hear what they was asking the other patient. You'd call and call for help to go to the bathroom but nobody come to take you. Or they give you a bedpan. You sitting on the bedpan on a cart, next to mens, crying for them to come. You were on the bed pan hurting because you were sitting on it so long."

She spoke of the lines in the County outpatient pharmacy. "You'd wait in line for hours until you are so tired you have to leave without your medications. I'd come back three days later and they still were not ready."

Ms. Windy C. recounted a recent visit to the County ER. Windy had first become my patient at County in the early 1980s when I was still in training. Over time, I became the doctor for her family, her four sisters and their children. Windy and I were the same age. When she arrived in Chicago from Birmingham, Alabama in 1964, Windy was twelve. County was their family's first hospital. They all came there. In her youth in Birmingham, Windy was a witness to, if not a direct participant in, the civil rights clashes of the era. The year before she and her family fled to the North four girls were killed in the 16th Street Baptist Church bombing. She witnessed the marches, and the arrest of Martin Luther King, the fire hosing of the children marchers, Bull Conner and his attack dogs. It was a frightening time but, unlike Ms. T who grew up in a more subservient time, Windy's attitudes were forged during this period. She was assertive and had no hesitation about speaking up if she thought something was wrong.

Today she was agitated as she spoke of her visit. She had retired from the Chicago Public Schools and had health insurance. But at $700 per month she could not always afford the additional co-pay for her medications. Hers was a common story. Many of our patients with good insurance could not afford the out-of-pocket costs of their illnesses. Windy had a bad headache and decided she would go to the County Emergency Room to get checked out and get her prescriptions filled. It was a mistake.

Back in the early 1990s, during the Clinton presidency, we all believed that health reform was around the corner. What would the County patients do we speculated? My colleague Gordy Schiff and I decided to ask them. We surveyed patients sitting in the waiting room of two of our clinics and posed different health insurance scenarios. The article we wrote was titled, "Voting with Their Feet" and appeared in the *American Journal of Public Health.* At that time seventy-five percent of the County patients said they would continue to get their care at County but, if free medications were provided, the percentage rose to eighty-five percent. Free medicines and free care were the major reason why patients put up with the indignity of County care. Less than twenty percent cited the quality of care as the reason why they came to County.

Windy's experience started off fine. After a long wait in the cavernous and modern waiting room of the new Hospital, she was called, and brought into a room. The doctor examined her and sent her for an X-ray. So far so good. This is where things began to unwind. After the X-ray was completed she was returned to the ER and the examination room was now occupied. Windy was kept on a gurney in the hallway. She's a big-boned woman, full-sized and round. The hospital gown, designed for a much smaller person barely covered her.

"I was in a gown and had nothing to cover my butt. I was out in front of the nurses' station. And I kept calling for help. They just ignored me. Pretended I was not there. They was sitting right there and did not come."

What pushed her over the top was the elderly lady, a stick-thin woman with worried eyes, who lay on the stretcher next to her. Windy struck up a conversation. The old lady had high blood pressure and had come to the Emergency Room because she had fallen down. Windy wondered if she had suffered a stroke. A nurse came to discharge her from the emergency room. The old lady protested, weakly.

"I can't stand. I'm afraid I'll fall."

"You have to go. The doctor says you're all right to leave," the nurse insisted. She was just following orders. The ER was packed with patients.

Windy jumped in, from the perch of her gurney, to defend the old lady, pulling the too-small blue hospital gown over her rear with one hand in an attempt to protect her modesty.

"She says she cannot walk! Why don't you listen to her? Can't you see she's sick? She's gonna fall! " she said, her voice rising in pitch and volume.

The nurse ignored her and helped the old woman get dressed and off the stretcher. The nurse was just doing her job. Not a bad person, just an ER nurse in the busiest ER in Cook County. More patients to see. The patient stood, tried to steady herself on the stretcher then collapsed like a rag doll to the floor.

Windy lost it. She screamed in frustration at the nurse. The nurse yelled back.

"I told you she was going to fall. Anyone could see that!" Windy said, her voice escalating to a shout.

The other people at the nurses' station paid no attention, as though this outburst was par for the course. Windy grabbed her clothes from under the head of the stretcher, as she cussed out the nurse and County. She dressed herself, using the gown as a partial screen on the stretcher in front of the nurses' triage area. She slid off the gurney and cursed at the staff as she tramped out, her finger wagging in rage at the nurses who sat behind the desk, impassive as statues.

"You know what you are? You all are bitches!" she said before she stormed off.

"I have not been that angry in years," she said to me as her fury at the reliving of this experience subsided. "I thought they would arrest me," she chuckled. "I ain't never going back there," she shook her wigged head. "Hm. Hm. Hm," she voiced her disgust. "They should have never let those people move into the new hospital."

The last recounting of a County Hospital experience by one of my patients was one that showed the potential for great service at County. This patient sustained a third degree burn to his leg in 2010 while at work. Employed and insured his whole adult life, he had heard stories about the poor customer service at County but had never been a patient there. He was referred to the outpatient burn clinic at County for treatment of his burn.

"I heard all the horror stories," he said, "but that has not been my experience. The care I received was great. Both by the staff and the doctors."

He told how he showed up thirty minutes before his appointment and was always seen at the specific appointment time as well as treated with respect and dignity.

Four anecdotes about County Hospital customer service from four patients that covered six decades, from the 1950s, when my first patient went to County, until 2010, when my last patient visited. While by no means a representative sample they reflected some truths about the system. The patients did and still experience indignities in the process of receiving treatment. While much had improved, the customer service was one aspect of County that never improved during my years there and still is a challenge today. The new hospital building eliminated many of structural deficiencies such as open wards that allowed for the humiliating patient experiences of which Mrs. T and Ms. NW spoke. But good customer service required more than just structural improvements.

Human dignity for our patients was at the core of our battles at County. All those years, all those meetings, all the programs we developed. We believed that our patients had the right to receive health care, but just as important, they should be treated like human beings. This was not just about external funding, overcrowding and political patronage—though these were major forces that detracted from our ability to provide the best service for the patients. It was not just about the doctors, the nurses and the administrators. Of all the challenges at the County Hospital, the delivery of respectful care to all the patients has been the most difficult to achieve on a consistent basis. We knew how to provide care once the patient arrived at our examination rooms. But we could not control what happened before or after. And sometimes the humiliating treatment the patients faced along the way sapped the spirits of the most resolute of our patients. One of our biggest failings was that we could not consistently improve the patient experience perceptions of our patients. Many of them, when they obtained health insurance, "voted with their feet" and went elsewhere.

Customer service is getting new attention since 2008 under the direction of the new County Health System Board of Directors. The crowd of patients who used to line up every day at 6:30 a.m., braving the elements while waiting to get into Fantus Clinic, has been moved inside. They still wait, but inside. At the Board's urging the County Health System management team initiated timed appointments for patients visiting specialists at County's Fantus Clinic, a first in the history of the hospital. It's a start, sixty years after Mrs. T's first visit to County; with a long way to go toward the day when all County patients would be treated like "human beings."

CHAPTER 19

AIDS and the Lessons Learned

HIS ROBIN'S EGG-BLUE EYES stared straight ahead as he girded himself to walk down the clinic hallway, a patient's chart in his hand. The glow from the overhead fluorescent bulbs cast a harsh glare on his sunken temples and eye sockets. His jaw was clenched, his skin was sallow and he had dark raccoon circles under his eyes. His short cropped hair had turned steel gray during recent months. His once military posture sagged under the weight of the illness. His clothes hung off his skeletal frame like he was a scarecrow. Every step was an ordeal. He was so focused on the act of walking, he did not notice me pass. He was using all he had left just to hobble down the hall. It had been like this for the last month. He was going downhill. Every disease had its own pace and rhythm. As a doctor I had seen the inexorable pace of diseases in my patients, but never in a colleague. I felt my gut twist every time I saw him.

Ron Sable and I saw patients in the same hallway of the General Medicine Clinic. We had been sharing this hallway for years. In happier times we would stop in the hall, between patients, and kibitz about County, my family or his lover, Joe. Now he was dying from AIDS, a cruel death sentence. He was near the end, yet came into work to see his patients, even though it sapped every last bit of his strength to do so. He had a dry cough. In a few weeks he would be diagnosed with TB and would end his practice.

I knew of Ron before I met him. In fact, he was one of the reasons my group from Syracuse came to Cook County. His picture was on the cover of a magazine that was delivered to our collective in Syracuse, just about the time we were exploring Cook County Hospital. The article described the internship he was sharing with another County Hospital resident. We were intrigued by the idea of doing a medical residency part-time and followed in Ron's footsteps.

I met Ron during my first visit to Cook County in 1977. He exuded a Midwest warmth and geniality that endeared him to others. Ron was seven years older than I. He was a conscientious objector during the Vietnam War, but rather than escape to Canada or do alternative service, Ron volunteered as a medic in Vietnam. The horror of this experience politicized him. He became a peace activist with the Vietnam Veterans Against the War and eventually found his way to medical school. Along the way he discovered that he was gay. Open and proud of his sexual orientation, he came to Chicago after medical school in Missouri to train at Cook County and explore gay life in the "Boystown" district on Chicago's North Side. Boystown became a magnet for young gay men from small farming towns and cities across the Midwest. As the gay rights movement of the 1970s began to bring homosexuality out of the closet, the neighborhood became the center of a nightclub and bath scene where gay men could openly display their sexuality.

Many years ahead of me in life experience, he was two years ahead in residency and our social spheres overlapped. He came to County because, like all of us, he believed that health care was a human right and no place exemplified this value as much as County. In 1983 the full brunt of the AIDS epidemic hit County. Ron partnered with Renslow Sherer, another doctor in our group, to create an outpatient clinic to see patients with AIDS after they were discharged from the hospital. The stigma that came with the diagnosis of AIDS was so strong that they named the clinic after themselves, the Sable-Sherer Clinic, rather than the disease.

The AIDS virus bludgeoned populations of gay men and intravenous drug users in U.S. cities with a vengeance in the early 1980s, devastating the gay community in Chicago. Legions of stick-thin gay men, who looked like starvation victims, walked the streets of Chicago, as they wasted away under the attack of the virus. There were no effective treatments. Ron and Renslow were two of the leading practitioners of outpatient HIV care in Chicago.

The epidemic had a political dimension as homophobic policies were proposed. It was the Reagan years and right-wing ideologues deemed that AIDS was God's punishment for homosexuals. Some called for quarantines. Others called for mandatory partner-tracking. Ron became an outspoken supporter of equal rights for gay people and against legislation that might stigmatize patients with HIV by requiring them to disclose their identities, and risk losing their jobs and health insurance. It was natural for Ron to move from peace activism to gay activism. Soon he was identified as one of the leaders of the expanding North Side Chicago gay community, a population forced out of the closet and into the public psyche by the AIDS epidemic.

In 1987, Ron was asked by the leadership of the gay community to run for alderman. If elected, he would be the first openly gay alderman in Chicago. His candidacy received national attention. Harvey Milk, the openly gay San Francisco supervisor, who was gunned down by a political opponent in 1979, galvanized the Chicago gay community to seek political power. Ron ran against the Chicago Democratic Machine candidate on a progressive platform, which included a strong gay rights platform. He continued to serve as a doctor at Cook County. He lost the election and another one four years later in 1991. His political campaigns brought his sexual orientation front and center and he had to endure threats and taunts as a result. Not once did he falter or shy away from leadership. In the end, he forced his opponent to adopt more gay friendly policies to keep his seat and helped to destigmatize gay life in Chicago.

In the late 1980s, Ron discovered that he, like many of his patients, was HIV positive. Over time, his muscular frame melted away, the pink of his cheeks paled, his gait slowed and his optimism faltered. He never complained and came to work until the time he could no longer dress himself and get out the door. His physician and nurse friends in the General Medicine Clinic bore witness to his fortitude as he struggled over his last few months of life. Ron, always putting others first, made appointments to come speak with all his friends before he died. He saw me in the hallway of the clinic on one of his better days in 1993. "Let's get together," he said. "Soon."

A few weeks later, he and I went to the County Hospital cafeteria to have a cup of coffee together. We chatted about County and Joe, his lover. We talked about his work and our friendship. It was light and chatty. He did not brook sympathy or pity. It was our last conversation and I knew when we parted that I would not speak to him again. A few months before Ron's death, an event was held at the South Shore Country Club with the vastness of Lake Michigan as a backdrop and over 500 friends showed up to pay tribute to him. All had been touched, as I had been, by his grace and strength. He died on December 30, 1993.

The AIDS epidemic, before the availability of life-prolonging drugs, ripped through communities, killing people like Ron in the prime of their lives. In the 1980s and 1990s we all lost friends to this epidemic. Losing Ron to AIDS was painful for me and all of the physicians in the General Medicine Division. He had dedicated his work-life fighting to maintain dignity for patients with the disease and now had succumbed to it himself. His quiet but forceful voice as a health care activist was silenced by AIDS and left a leadership gap in the progressive gay community that was hard to fill.

However, others picked up his mantle. It did not take long for AIDS to move from being a disease of gay white men to becoming a disease of minority populations in the most devastated neighborhoods in the city. Misinformation about AIDS prevention in the community, fanned by inept and ideologically driven public-health messaging by the Reagan administration that emphasized "just say no" over condoms and needle-exchange programs, helped expand the epidemic.

Mardge Cohen's program for women and children with HIV was a national model for care for HIV-positive women and children. Mardge was a swirl of energy and New York intensity. Petite, powerful and prickly, she and her husband, Gordy Schiff, cut a contrasting swath as they walked the halls of County. He was tall, cordial and cerebral. She was short and brusque. You often heard her high-pitched voice echo off the walls before she emerged into view. Mardge was a champion of women's health issues, critical of authority and intolerant of injustice. People were split about her. Her intensity and sharp tongue alienated some. Others had a deep affection for her ability to speak the truth and her deep empathy for the plight of our patients.

The program that Mardge created was rooted in beliefs we all shared about health and medicine. First, we believed that decent health care was a right and our patients, especially our patients, deserved the best. Next, we believed the medical model of disease we had been taught was incomplete. Disease was viewed as something that emanated from the individual. While we all loved the practice of medicine, we took a public health perspective on disease and its causes. We saw disease as a manifestation of dysfunction at the level of family, community and society. Social injustice was as important a cause of disease as was biology. We had all gathered at the County Hospital in part because we shared this world view about the social determinants of disease and health.

Our beliefs originated from the perspective that if we were serious about improving health outcomes, we needed to focus our work on communities and society. In the spirit of the nineteenth-century German pathologist, Rudolf Virchow, we believed that politics was health care on a larger scale and that to improve health in Chicago we had to be politically engaged locally and nationally. On the personal level, we hoped always to approach the health of our patients from a perspective of curiosity, not judgment, about their lives and situations. Many of us were from backgrounds different from our patients. How could we possibly understand the struggles our patients faced? Finally, we gravitated toward inclusive approaches to care delivery, ones that were multidisciplinary and collective.

The Women and Children's Program that Mardge created in 1988 was one of the first comprehensive programs in the U.S. for women and children with HIV. By the late 1980s the rates of AIDS were rising in women. Their disease was more likely than not heterosexually transmitted and then vertically transmitted to their children. Mardge framed AIDS in women and children as a social issue; not a transmission issue. Women with AIDS tended to be marginalized and disempowered, often in abusive relationships, drug-addicted, or both. She realized that like all mothers, women with AIDS would care for their children first and for themselves last. She built the program as a place where women, their partners and their children could get all of their needs met in one place. It was a team-and-family-centered approach to care. As women got ill, the program helped them to address painful issues such as writing wills and providing for guardianship for their children. Mardge was able to pull together teams of physicians, nurses, and psychologists to create the support and services needed for these vulnerable individuals. She built a peer-to-peer counseling program that allowed women to break out of the isolation and demoralization that the disease and their drug addiction engendered. To provide the services, Mardge had to scrounge, cajole and write grants. She had few permanent staff to run the program. It angered her that exemplary care for these women and children had to be funded by grants instead of being supported by budgeted positions.

In the earliest days of the program, the women and their providers were crowded into the Radiation Center. It was an area located in an annex off the beaten path in Fantus Clinic, which was not designed as a clinical space. Some say that it was the original location of the Greek restaurant before it moved across the street to Pasteur Park. Regardless, it was not a real clinic space, but it was all that Mardge could find. And she made it work. It looked like a triage station on a battlefield, with providers kneeling down in the waiting area, as they spoke to clients who sat packed into chairs, row upon row. Voices bounced off

the walls. Children were playing in the hallways. Folks were standing in every spare space because there were too few seats. But Mardge
and her colleagues provided exceptional care. Her patients overlooked
the dismal surroundings because of the care they were receiving and
because, in many ways like most of our patients, they did not realize
that they could expect better.

By the early 1990s the growth and excellence of the AIDS clinical services at County, including the Women and Children's Program,
were recognized by County's leadership. County Hospital, in partnership with Rush University Medical Center, built a new treatment facility for patients living with HIV and AIDS. The Ruth M.
Rothstein Core Center, one of the largest and most beautiful AIDS
treatment centers in the country, now treats over thirty percent of the
HIV/AIDS patients in the city of Chicago.

Over time, the leadership of these clinical programs that made
Cook County Hospital the center for care of people with HIV in
Chicago was transferred to others. But the principles that guided the
care for patients with HIV/AIDS at the Core Center came directly
from the beliefs and politics of Ron, Mardge and Renslow: that health
care is a right; that illness or fear of illness should not be used to
limit the civil rights of patients with AIDS; that comprehensive care
needs to be dignified as well as family-and-community-oriented; that
the spread of diseases such as AIDS is caused by societal dysfunction
such as poverty, homophobia, racism and male chauvinism as much
as by the HIV virus; that other supportive services such as psychoso-
cial support, housing and food are as necessary a part of treatment as
medications; that research should be participatory and respectful. As
a measure of the enduring legacy of the founding philosophy of care
developed by the program founders, the CORE Center boasts the best
patient satisfaction scores in the County Health System.

In 2004, Mardge responded to a call from community organizations in Rwanda to help women infected with HIV as a result of the
genocide there in 1994. Women who were infected with HIV as a
result of rapes during the genocide were now getting ill and had few

health care resources. Mardge went to Rwanda and in collaboration with community groups created a program called We-Actx for women and families living with HIV/AIDS in Kigali, based on the program she had created in Chicago. Many of the problems facing women with HIV/AIDS in Kigali were similar to those women faced in Chicago. And the Kigali program addressed not only clinical care but family support, nutrition and job creation. The spirit of Ron Sable lived on long after his death, in the work of Mardge Cohen and others, halfway around the world from the clinic he had founded more than twenty years earlier.

CHAPTER 20

Crossing the Threshold

"YOU SHOULDN'T LEAVE, DAVID" she said, her Brooklyn-accented voice permeating the room. My eyes widened. I stood in her office in front of her desk. She sat, like an empress in her chair—the CEO of the Cook County Bureau of Health Services. I felt like a field mouse in her presence. Her blue eyes, sharp nose and regal gaze made her look like a bird of prey. She did not miss a thing.

"There are others here who should leave." She listed the names of my friends. "But you, David." She paused and wagged her finger for emphasis, "You should not leave."

I had come to tell her that I had been offered the job of Chairman of Medicine at Mount Sinai Hospital, her former institution, and asked her thoughts. She was perturbed, not pleased by my revelation. She was a hard woman to please. I felt awkward, like a schoolboy in her presence and shuffled my feet from side to side.

"But, David. You have to do what's best for you."

Ruth Rothstein was tall and imperious with a ramrod bearing. She was dressed to the nines. Her hair was perfectly coiffed, each one in its place. Power emanated from her like Chanel No. 5. Her reputation had preceded her arrival at County. She had been the Chief Executive Officer at Mount Sinai Hospital in Chicago for nineteen years, a hospital that everyone agreed should not still be open. It was the same hospital that was recruiting me to come lead the Department of

Internal Medicine. Despite my feelings of intimidation, truth be told, I liked Ruth. And I did not want her to hear of my recruitment from someone else.

The general opinion was that Mrs. Ruth Rothstein was responsible for the survival of that hospital located just a mile or so away from Cook County in the impoverished North Lawndale community of Chicago. Once home to a thriving Jewish population of 120,000 people, between 1950 and 1960 all the white people moved out and 120,000 black people from the South moved in while panic-peddling real estate brokers exploited racial fears. When white flight occurred, the physician base of the hospital eroded and the growth of the uninsured imperiled its existence.

Ruth grew up in New York, graduated from high school and began to work as a labor organizer for the Union of Electrical Workers. She moved to Chicago to organize and eventually became an evening lab technician in a Chicago hospital. Before long she was running the lab. She moved to Mount Sinai Hospital in 1968 and worked her way up to be the special assistant to the CEO. When he was fired by the Board in 1972, Ruth became President and CEO of the hospital, one of the few women CEOs (other than nuns) running a major Chicago hospital. It was like taking over command of the *Titanic* after it hit the iceberg. And in an environment of sexism, plate-glass ceilings and low prospects for women in the 1970s, Ruth succeeded beyond anyone's expectations and to some folks' dismay.

Using common sense, a network of personal relationships and the power of her personality, Ruth guided that hospital through three of the most turbulent decades in U.S. health care. In 1968, the death of Martin Luther King spurred riots in Chicago and the West Side went up in flames. Most of the Jewish businesses that lined Roosevelt Road near the hospital were burned out and looted. Federal troops were camped out in Douglas Park across from the hospital. Prior to this time there were smatterings of patients who would come from other neighborhoods to Sinai for care. After the riots, almost none came.

The hospital hobbled along for the next four years trying to maintain the original Jewish, insured patient base. But in 1972, the Board was faced with a dilemma. Should Mount Sinai abandon Lawndale and move to a new facility in the northern suburbs where the Jewish population had moved? Ruth presented the options to the Board.

"But," she warned, "if you decide that Mount Sinai stays, then you have to make a commitment to this community and its needs." The Board decided to stay put and Ruth guided Sinai Hospital to become a key link in the safety-net hospital network, both in Chicago and nationally. Long on the top of the list of endangered Chicago hospitals at risk for extinction, Sinai always survived. Down went Saint Anne's, Roosevelt, Augustana and eleven others. There were two historically Jewish hospitals in Chicago in the 1970s. The wealthy one, Michael Reese Hospital, on the swanky lakeshore, founded by urbane German Jews in the 1850s, was one of the premier teaching hospitals in the country. Then there was Mount Sinai, founded by shtetl-born, Eastern European Jews in 1919, in the Jewish West Side ghetto. One the jewel of the crown, the other a tow-headed stepchild. From the earliest days Sinai tottered on the verge of closing. In 2010, only Mount Sinai was still open. Ruth won the American Hospital Association's Hospital Administrator of the Year Award in testimony to her stewardship of Sinai through these years.

But you did not want to be on her bad side. One of my colleagues told me the following story of Ruth visiting the office of Big Jim Thompson, Republican Governor of Illinois in the 1980s. A group of hospital CEOs asked to meet the Governor, who had begun a program that limited Medicaid payments to safety-net hospitals, imperiling their balance sheets. A deputy to the Governor met with them and gave a wonky and long winded speech on the intricacies of the state budget and the Governor's priorities, which did not include Medicaid expansion. The CEOs listened in polite silence. Ruth seethed. Unable to take it anymore, Ruth stood up and interrupted the bureaucrat mid-sentence with an order. "Shut up!"

She approached his desk like a gunslinger and leaned over him, as he stared up in disbelief. "You see these keys?" A set of keys dangled and clinked from her index finger in front of his face. Her red nail polish glittered. She was going into her windup. "These are the keys to Mount Sinai Hospital. If you don't give us more money, I can't run Mount Sinai Hospital." She slammed the keys down on the walnut desk in front of the Governor's aide and pointed her finger at him. "So, since you are so smart, you can run the fucking hospital." She turned and stormed out of the Executive Suite. Her shoes clickity-clacked down the corridor. The other hospital CEOs stared in silence as the Governor's aide jumped up from his desk and chased Ruth down the hallway. He brought her back to the office, asked the other CEOs to leave and made a deal with her to send more state money to Mount Sinai. Probably this story, like a fine cheese, had ripened with time but such was the power of Ruth thirty years later, that these fables of her influence still had legs.

When Ruth was recruited from Sinai to come to lead County in 1991, the hospital was on the ropes. Since the county government usurped control in 1979 the hospital had deteriorated. County had been disaccredited for fire safety and other problems and had suffered through a series of political hacks and incompetent leaders whose only talent seemed to be patronage hiring. Ruth was the first professional hospital administrator in decades. She wasted no time in cleaning up the place and creating a sense of optimism about the future.

Ruth's strategy for building the new hospital was straightforward. She positioned herself at the center of the campaign. She assembled a civic coalition of some of the most prominent A-list individuals in Chicago to get them behind a new hospital. After months of tours of the old hospital and meetings with editorial boards, the corner was turned. She finally even managed to flip the *Tribune* after it had been railing for years against the rebuilding of County. At last, the *Tribune* wrote an editorial that supported the new County Hospital. Years of demonstrations and strikes, against all odds, with a wall of opposition from the *Tribune*, the private hospitals and most of Chicago's political leadership were over. Most opposition was vanquished. There was going to be a new County Hospital. Ruth Rothstein had pushed, nudged and prodded until she got what we all wanted and the patients needed—a new County Hospital.

The mid-1990s were the best they had been at County since I arrived in 1978. I was Chief of the General Internal Medicine and Primary Care Division. I took this position after leaving the walk-in-clinic. Our Division had grown from the original ten primary care physicians in the early 1980s to over fifty. In addition to a new County Hospital, the plans to create an ambulatory care network and expand primary care into the community were well under way. It was a watershed time and a vindication of our belief that a regional primary care network linked to the hospital was a crucial component of the County system. The Core Center for the treatment of AIDS was being planned in partnership with Rush-Presbyterian. Even the conditions for the doctors in training improved. All the inpatients were seen by attending physicians who helped manage the patient care decisions. The residents in this era had much more supervision and the care of the patients improved as a result. A far cry from the wild and crazy times during our residencies. It was a time of heady optimism at County. So why was I standing in Ruth's office and talking of leaving?

It was the phone call from Sinai that stirred the pot. "Would you interview for the job of Chairman of Medicine here?" Before this call, I had never considered leaving County. I was a lifer. One by one, my friends from medical school had left County before me. Jim Schlosser had moved to Boston. The others had left as well. I was the last one left from the "Syracuse Group." I was forty-two years old. I loved the challenge of practicing medicine in an underserved community and it brought me great satisfaction to work at County. I was attracted to the intractable, to problems no one wanted to tackle. I enjoyed the complexity of trying to improve broken systems of care. But I had never worked anywhere but County. I began to think back on my accidental career there. I had thought I would stay for four years and then go back East. Now it was almost seventeen years. I was curious about

Sinai. Here was a system that served the poor as well. It was deeply rooted to the Lawndale community. Despite the optimism of the times, there was still much dysfunction at County Hospital—despite our best efforts to serve our patients. It unsettled me. Problems with access to key services. The poor service the patients received. Was Berwick correct? Was County designed to give the results we actually got? Was a system whose purpose was to serve the poor destined to perpetuate separate and unequal care despite our best efforts to transform it? Despite the new administration, we had never overcome the corrosive influence of politics and patronage, the terrible customer service, the lack of basic supplies and slow services that contributed to poorer outcomes.

We were proud of the care we delivered. A report in the *Chicago Tribune* in the mid 1980s stated that County Hospital had the second lowest mortality rate of the 100 hospitals surveyed. This was the irony of County. It was possible to deliver really good care. But the systemic barriers that kept patients from getting the care they needed on time had never been resolved from the earliest days of the hospital. Underfunding was a problem. But there was more than just funding that was the problem. There needed to be a "cultural revolution" at the County Hospital, where all patients could expect to be treated with respect and dignity. This culture of service was not ingrained in the hospital and clinics and contributed to negative patient experiences.

Something inside me said it was time to leave. There were things I could learn if I left County that I could not learn there. I thought ahead. In the future, with some experience gained outside of County, maybe I could return, follow in the footsteps of Quentin Young and contribute to a transformation that would finally realize the potential of the place.

When I was called and asked to interview for the position of Chairperson of Medicine at Mount Sinai Hospital, I decided to check it out. It was not an easy job. An urban teaching hospital, in one of the poorest neighborhoods in Chicago, it floundered on the edge of bankruptcy. After Ruth Rothstein left, everyone thought the axe would drop and it would be shuttered. But Benn Greenspan, Ruth's second-in-command and now CEO, had managed to get the Board and the medical staff behind him and the hospital stumbled along. Ruth reiterated her advice to me.

"David, you have to do what is best for you and your family."

What's best for me? It was one of the most difficult decisions of my life. I felt like a teenager leaving home for the first time. Everything that I had learned about being a doctor I had learned at County. It was my first and only job as a doctor. I had the County bug. How was I going to leave the place that had been my home for the past seventeen years? My friends thought I was nuts to leave. County, with all its problems, was at least funded by tax dollars. Sinai, had no such safetynet. Barack Obama, who was Chairman of the Illinois State Senate Health Committee before he became U.S. Senator, was a frequent visitor to Sinai. Once he wisecracked, "Saving Sinai is a full-time job." A colleague left a *Chicago Sun Times* on my desk. The front page headline screamed, "Sinai to Close." The story quoted Benn Greenspan, the Sinai CEO, predicting that the hospital would close if the State of Illinois did not give more money. It was a story that would play out over and over during my time there. But front page news about a failing inner city hospital did not deter me. Not after what I had been through. It was time for me to leave County.

My father, who had been so supportive of my going to County from medical school, seventeen years earlier, encouraged me to take the job. He was in the hospital, suffering from what was to be his terminal illness. I brought my contract from Sinai with me to his hospital room and had a brief discussion about the job. He had no doubts. He died three weeks before I started my new position.

I was dazed for months. The loss of my dad *and* leaving County was more than I could manage. I kept my emotions bottled inside as I boxed up my office at County, throwing out papers I had hoarded since medical school. For the first few weeks on the new job, my car would drive to the County exit off the Eisenhower and I would sheepishly circle back and drive down Ogden Avenue to Sinai. Sometimes, when I was in the neighborhood, I would walk around the block or enter the front lobby of the old hospital for old time's sake. A booster dose. But never once did I forget what County had given me. To this day, any time, day or night, when driving down the Eisenhower, it does not matter what I am doing, when I whizz past the shuttered, old County Hospital, I always turn to look.

CHAPTER 21

1995: 'Til Death Do We Part

DURING THESE YEARS I CONTINUED to see patients. In my seventeen years at County and then at Sinai, I kept my primary care practice. As a primary care doctor, I had taken care of three generations of Chicago families and had a front-row seat into their lives. They had put their trust in me. I had done my best to manage their illnesses and guide them through troubled times. They had counseled me too. If primary care was an immersion experience, after thirty years, I was soaked.

I first encountered Harriet B. in my clinic in the summer of 1978, my internship year. She was radiant with a wide smile, coffee complexion and large clear light brown eyes.

"Hi, I'm Doctor Ansell, pleased to meet you."

"I'm Harriet B.," she responded and relayed her story in a soft voice. She was thirty-four years old, just eight years older than I. She had sickle cell anemia and an ulcer on her left foot. It was very painful and she wanted my help. I had only seen sickle cell anemia patients when they were admitted to the hospital screaming and writhing in pain. Until Harriet walked in I never treated a patient with the disease in the office. I was a novice.

She was pale, consistent with chronic anemia. The whites of her eyes had a faint orange-yellow glow, the sign of active destruction of her red blood cells as is common with this disease. Her heart pounded and I heard a whooshing murmur through my stethoscope, another sign of severe anemia. And on her left ankle bone she had a large ulcer the size of a grapefruit. I put some gloves on and examined it. She grimaced in pain. I had never seen anything like this. She had had it for a few years. Every treatment had failed.

After she dressed, we sat and talked. I bared my soul. "Mrs. B.," I said, "I have taken care of some patients with sickle cell anemia in the hospital, but I am not experienced with treating foot ulcers. I can do some asking around and if you come back in a month I should have some answers." She had probably waited for hours to see me today. To get the appointment at Fantus, she had probably waited months. I offered her my earnest inexperience, which was not much solace. She had probably been hoping for one of the County superdocs, one of the "best doctors" they spoke of. Instead she landed me. "That's all right, Dr. Ansell," she let me off the hook, "I'll come back in a month." And that is how a twenty-six year relationship began.

The next month I was armed with answers. I had read some articles and consulted with the plastic surgeons. We first had to debride the ulcer—scrape all the dead tissue off until the ulcer was hamburger red. I showed Harriet how to do it. Over the next few months we worked to get the ulcer clean. Then a skin graft. I admitted Harriet to the hospital to get a blood transfusion before the graft because this had been shown to improve the healing. The skin graft took and the pain was gone.

As the years passed, she relied on me more and more as complications of the disease progressed: she had a gall bladder attack; surgery; then a stroke; partial blindness; and multiple hospitalizations for transfusions and for painful bone attacks. I was a witness to all of these complications. I saw her every hospitalization. In twenty-six years she was hospitalized over 200 times, usually for a week at a time, almost four years of hospital sojourns; plus monthly visits to my office. We got to know each other pretty well. Along the way the formalities were dropped. I called her Harriet. She called me David.

The jarring ring of the phone rousted me from my deep sleep. Half-awake, I grasped for the receiver and brought it to my ear. "Hello," I said, as I forced my blinking eyes open to the pitch-black of the bedroom. I glanced at my alarm clock on the nightstand next to the phone. It was hours before dawn. Paula was deep asleep beside me.

Silence. Only rapid, short panting transmitted through the receiver, like Morse Code. I shook myself wide awake.

"Harriet?" I whispered, "Is that you?"

No answer. "Harriet?" I asked.

"Yes, David." I could barely hear her voice above the rapid panting. I had learned to read her voice. Control was important to her. She never cried or showed emotion. I imagined her stone-faced clenched jaw on the other side of the phone.

"How do you feel?" I asked. A stupid question. The fact of the phone call was all the information I needed. She called only when her pain was spiraling out of control.

"David, I'm hurting," she said. Her rapid panting said it all.

"Have Bill bring you to the hospital," I said. "I'll call ahead." I knew what was coming next.

"I don't want to go to the hospital," she said. Harriet had a post traumatic stress reaction to the hospital. She suffered teeth-grinding pain until it twisted her into submission. She despised the hospital.

"Harriet, you need to come in now," I said. "I'll take care of you."

"Okay," she replied. "But not to the Emergency Room." More than the inpatient units Harriet hated the Emergency Room. She had been a patient in Chicago hospital ERs hundreds of times and the experience was degrading. By her mid-forties, she refused to go. Late at night in the grit of a Chicago trauma ER, the knife and gunshot wounds had priority. They screamed in pain. Blood and chaos. The drunks and the addicts on gurneys as well. Harriet was a hapless witness, her chest and legs wracked with electric shocks of pain. She waited in vain for relief. Harriet did not rock and scream when she was in crisis. Instead, she lay very still and silent, like a baby bird that had fallen out of her nest, her eyes wide open and pupils dilated in agony and in fear, her rapid breathing and pulse the only clues to her distress. Doctors and nurses would assume, in their inexperience or stupidity, that she was drug-seeking, because she did not writhe and cry like the others. They would never give her enough pain medication. Or they delayed her treatment because she did not look sick.

So Harriet decided she had had enough. The only way Harriet would come to the hospital was if she could go directly to the medical floor and be treated there, by me and my team.

"OK, Harriet, I'll admit you to the hospital. I'll call ahead and let them know you are coming. Have Bill take you to Admitting."

Sickle cell anemia is a genetic disease caused by a substitution of one nucleotide for another in the DNA of the affected individual, causing the red blood cells to twist into abnormal sickle shapes under stressful situations. If the defect was hidden in the DNA of the mother's and the father's genes, then the child of that union had a one in four chance of getting the full-blown disease. In the United States, it was a disease of black people.

Sickle cell anemia was first described in the scientific literature in 1910. Ironically, that first description had a County Hospital connection. A medical student from Trinidad who was training at County Hospital in the early 1900s had symptoms of undiagnosed sickle cell anemia and went to see Dr. James Herrick, a famous Rush physician, who looked at his blood under a microscope and described his findings in the *Journal of the American Medical Association*. It took 300 years after the arrival of the first slave ships for this disease to be described, despite the fact that it was present in black people in the United States during that entire period. It is a testimony to the sheer power of slavery and racism that such a striking and violent illness defied discovery in the U.S. until Herrick.

Sickle cell disease devastates. The sickling of the red blood cells is the cause of most of the complications of the disease. These sickled blood cells clog up the small blood vessels of the body—slamming off the supply of blood and slowly killing tissues, bit by bit. Most patients with this disease are dead by the age of forty, with destruction to their organs caused by the abnormal blood cells. The heart, lung, kidneys, brain and other vital organs are all affected. One of the most disturb-

ing complications the patients experience is pain, bone breaking, like
nails hammered into the bones.

When a sickled blood cell traverses a small artery in the bones of a
patient, it chokes the vessel, causing a decreased blood flow to a small
area of bone. The bone infarcts and dies. The pain is so excruciating
that the patient rocks, writhes back and forth and screams until relief
comes in the form of narcotics. The pain attacks are associated with
weather changes or viral infections, but when the pain descends, there
is no stopping it.

I walked onto the hospital unit and into Harriet's room. She lay
motionless in the hospital bed. Intravenous saline dripped in her arm.
On the bedside stand was a phone. The overhead bedside light highlighted her big brown eyes, jaundiced from the destruction of red
blood cells. She was perfectly still. Only her eyes moved to acknowledge my presence. Her lip quivered. Pain. She did not speak. It was
too much effort, a sign of the bone-cracking pain she was experiencing. A less-experienced observer might think she was resting
peacefully.

"Hi, Harriet, how's the pain?" I always called ahead to the hospital
and tried to speak with the residents and the floor nurses, to explain
that Harriet was not a malingerer, that her silence indicated pain. But
the culture of suspicion was too hard to eradicate, and she was mis-
treated by someone during a hospitalization. Someone accused her of
craving drugs, or held back the narcotics.

"Not good, David," she whispered.

I raised her dose of medication. I knew that I had treated her
enough when she finally fell asleep.

Bill, Harriet's husband, was a cab driver, a brawny, muscled, working-class man, tough and gruff. Bill mistrusted doctors and hospitals,
and he defended Harriet with an in-your-face intensity.

"They are not treating her right," Bill said to me as we stood on
the hospital floor just outside her hospital room. "That's wrong, man.
That's just wrong."

His coal-colored eyes held my gaze as his voice boomed down the floor, attracting glances from nurses and visitors. I listened in sympathy and waited until he was finished. He was angry and his voice expanded the more enraged he became. People could mistake his anger for aggression. But he was upset for good reason. Bill hated to see Harriet in pain and his exasperation grew from his love for her. Maybe nineteen or twenty years into her illness, he began to take a more active role. Bill was much more intolerant of the failings of our hospital care delivery system than his wife. After I left County and moved to Sinai, Harriet, who had followed me there, had yet another episode of hospitalization for pain during which she was accused of wanting too much pain medication. Bill blew his top again.

It was time for an intervention. I asked Bill and Harriet to come in and speak to the nursing staff and the house staff about Harriet's experiences as a patient and Bill's experience as a family member. The house staff and nursing staff sat in chairs in the hospital conference room. Harriet, Bill and I sat in the center. I told the staff the reason for the meeting. Years of frustration and disappointment poured out as Bill and Harriet portrayed their experience with the medical care system first at County and next at Sinai.

Harriet talked about her fears. It began in childhood with frantic trips to the hospital. Her pain was not acknowledged by the hospital staff through all these years. How all the sad memories of past mistreatment and humiliation bubbled up and were re-experienced by her at each crisis, a post-traumatic stress experience; how she feared coming to the hospital; how she had learned to lie still and not cry when she was in pain; how she was a mother and a churchgoing lady but was treated like a drug addict.

Bill was riled, but in control. "Do you think she wants to come to the hospital?" He asked. "How do you think she feels when you accuse her of being a drug addict? How would you respond if it was your wife or husband?" He fired off these questions with machine-gun rapid fire. The nurses and house staff listened and asked questions.

It worked. Harriet began to receive better care. After one hospitalization, almost twenty years into our relationship, Harriet stopped walking, a neuromuscular complication of the short-acting narcotic she received. A known side effect, it frightened her. With physical therapy, her strength returned, but I had to find a new way to treat her. I did some reading. I had been treating her pain incorrectly. For twenty years. As an intern, I had learned the treatment for sickle pain from the residents who came before me in residency. We all learned the same way. Then I passed it down to generations of other doctors, only to discover that it was dead wrong. The short-acting narcotic we used had to be given at least every two hours to be effective. On the floors that interval was impossible for the nurses to handle. So the gap between dosages went to four and then six hours. Too long. By then the pain had built to a crescendo and was difficult to control. What if we could treat her with long-acting narcotics that she could control herself through an intravenous pump? If she felt a wave of pain she could self-administer the medication. Overnight, we switched the way we treated pain, not just for Harriet but for all patients with chronic pain at the hospital. The medication I had been using for twenty years was taken off the formulary so it could not be ordered. I encouraged Harriet to call me sooner, before her pain became unbearable, and I admitted her directly to a hospital bed rather than have her come through the emergency room. I left orders for the residents and nurses to initiate the new treatment. Overnight, Harriet's hospitalizations were shorter and the pain controlled more quickly.

Eventually, the toll of the illness broke her body down—piece by piece, organ by organ. Her cocoa-colored complexion darkened to steel black from the years of stress and from iron deposits from hundreds of blood transfusions. The whites of her eyes turned muddy ochre and sank into her face. Dark raccoon rings circled them. They looked like miners headlamps against her now gaunt and wrinkled face. Her hair, once a luxuriant brown, morphed into an iron-gray halo of brittle Brillo above her head. Her heart failed. Then her liver. Every step sapped her breath and flared her nostrils. The periods between her painful episodes became shorter and shorter until chronic pain settled in her bones like a cancer. She required long-acting narcotics all the time. She hobbled into my office and with each zombie step gritted her teeth.

The vise tightened when her kidneys failed. She never wanted to go on kidney dialysis. Bill's brother had been a dialysis patient and Harriet expressed her fear of it. She was once again in a hospital bed, dying. Her arms and legs twitched from the lethal poisons that accumulated in her blood from her failing kidneys. The end was near. It was time for a decision.

Bill and I stood by Harriet's bedside. The light from the afternoon sky streamed through her hospital window and lit up her bed. We discussed her options: no kidney dialysis and a certain and painless death within the next two weeks; kidney dialysis and life constrained by pain and ultimate liver or other organ failure. Bill and Harriet were grandparents. Harriet had brought her granddaughter to the clinic, a chubby little girl with pigtails. She had Harriet's eyes and smile. They doted on her. Bill had been vehement in his opposition to dialysis. But now facing the end he looked at me and queried, "Why not choose life?" Bill loved Harriet and could not bear to lose her. Harriet's eyes were wide open and clear. A moment of lucidity from the soporific, noxious swill of renal toxins.

"What do you think, David?" she asked, as she struggled to get the words out. I could barely hear her. A few towels and a mustard colored plastic wash basin were piled on the ledge next to the bed, under the window. The TV was murmuring in the background, a mindless soap opera. I had been Harriet's doctor for most of my adult life. She would face a life of pain and disability on dialysis. She had aged so much that the doctors and nurses thought Bill was her son. But in his eyes, she was still the beautiful young woman he had married years before. She too had reasons to keep living. I did not want to lose her either.

"Choose life," I agreed.

We started dialysis. Harriet lived two more years. When she died I delivered a eulogy at her funeral at a storefront Baptist church on Chicago's South Side. The sun peeked through the windows of the one-room church and dappled the room with light. Wooden pews faced a raised stage with a wood lectern in the middle. On the right side of the stage there was a drum set and a small electric organ. Three middle-aged men in suits climbed to the stage, one carrying an electric guitar. Soon the small room was oscillating with gospel singing and clapping. At the end of the service, the pastor called me up. As the musicians played in the background, I climbed the steps to the pulpit and grabbed the wooden edges of the lectern to steady myself. Bill and Harriet's son sat in the audience with twenty or so family members and church members. They swayed to the rhythm. I spoke about the strength of a woman through a lifetime of illness, about the love between a man and his wife, about the decision to choose life, and about a doctor who lost his patient and friend.

CHAPTER 22

2002: Last Rounds

Wᴀᴛ ᴋɪɴᴅ ᴏꜰ ꜰᴀʀᴇᴡᴇʟʟ do you give a condemned building? One whose doors should have been shuttered seventy years ago? Perhaps, an arson's torch should have put it out of its misery. Let the world forget the wretchedness that filled the wards of this godforsaken place. Instead, we had a party. Only Gordy Schiff could have pulled this off.

Gordy Schiff had been a fixture at County since 1969 when he volunteered in the emergency room as a college student. Tall and spindly like a sun-starved beanstalk, he was ill-kempt in a mad scientist sort of way. His clothes did not quite fit his frame, his sandy hair shagged over his ears and neck and his sideburns were a throwback to 1968. Gordy was the resident intellectual and eccentric of our group. His office resembled the apartment of the neighborhood recluse, teeming with file cabinets and piles upon piles of papers and journal articles.

Gordy was a pack rat—he hoarded medical journal articles and Neil Young tracks. He described himself once as "an obsessive compulsive off the deep end." Long after many of us had trashed our paper files in favor of internet searching, Gordy maintained his reams of catalogued papers. He liked the feel of paper in his hands, much as a rare book librarian revels in the tactile delight of the parchment of ancient tomes. But despite the appearance of disarray and distraction, Gordy reached into a pile of papers with a cheery "I have it here somewhere" and produced the paper that had just been referenced by him, without skipping a beat. He had his quirky rules which he insisted you learned as well. A two-page article was never stapled. Never. Gordy used a small piece of scotch tape to hold these together. For larger papers only a Bostitch stapler worked. He was so enamored of Bostitch staplers, that he bought them and gave them away at his retirement party. *Swingline* was anathema. When it came to staplers, Gordy was a dilettante.

Recently, a famous infectious disease doctor died and his obituary was highlighted in the *New York Times*. I remembered where I stood, as a young resident when Gordy gave me the first article I had read by this doctor. In the absence of attending physicians, residents like Gordy were our lifeline to medical knowledge during our training. Even today, I turn to him when I have an arcane question about a paper in medicine.

Gordy was curious about the innate workings of hospitals that made things unsafe for patients. A disciple of Edward Deming and Avedis Donabedian, quality improvement gurus, he chaired the quality committee in the Department of Medicine at County Hospital for twenty years. One famous Deming quote, "Every defect is a treasure," was Gordy's mantra. He was a specialist in identifying defects. Like a medical etymologist, he found defects in common medical practices. A savant in the field of quality and safety, years before the patient safety movement took hold in the country, he asked simple questions like: "Why can't our computer system that prescribed medications communicate with our computer systems that reported laboratory tests?" He looked at abnormal laboratory tests to see if patients had been contacted. He measured the added value that an attending physician made to inpatient rounds. He became a national expert on errors doctors made in diagnosing illness. He was a passionate opponent of Big Pharma and its influence on the prescribing behavior of physicians. The *Physician's Desk Reference* (PDR) is a Pharma compilation that was at one time sent annually to all doctors in the U.S. free of charge. Every doctor's office in the U.S. had at least one copy. Once Gordy, on one of his campaigns, took a red magic marker and wrote "BAD BOOK" in large letters on all the *PDRs* he found in the General Medicine Clinic at County.

The systems at County were often so screwed up that Gordy became an expert in broken systems and how to diagnose the problems. There was a lot that went wrong around us that required thinking about things in new ways. Gordy once said to me about County, "At County we are so far behind, we are ahead." He was right.

Gordy was dismissed as a gadfly by successive department chairs and hospital administrations and never got the local respect that his prodigious talents deserved. But sometimes through Gordy's sheer will and good-natured persistence, the bureaucrats relented and let him solve a problem. In 2006, the outpatient pharmacy at the Fantus Clinic collapsed into a dysfunctional funk so severe that the patient wait for prescriptions went from hours to weeks. It was so bad that it made the front page of the *Chicago Tribune*, as another example of County Hospital ineptitude. Desperate, the hospital administration turned to Gordy, who fixed the problem.

It surprised no one when Gordy proposed a day to honor the history of the old Cook County Hospital, shortly before the opening of the replacement hospital we had all worked so hard to see. In true Burnham Chicago tradition to "make no small plans," Gordy proposed "Last Rounds." His scheme was bold and captured the imagination of the hospital staff: send out invitations to all the doctors who had ever trained at County; invite them to return to Chicago and meet at the County Hospital on a Saturday; arrange for a legion of students to record and document the scene; have the doctors gather in the solaria, the windowed south-facing tips of the long patient care wards, in the main hospital building and share remembrances of County. This would be followed by a tour of the soon-to-open new County Hospital, seventy four years after the American College of Surgeons called for the building of a new facility.

It was a crazy idea, but Gordy pulled it off. On a sunny fall morning in 2002, doctors from all over the U.S. gathered at old Cook County Hospital and registered. They ranged in age from 92 to their early thirties. I had been away from County for six years. As I walked down the hallway of Ward 24, past the yellow tile walls, the nursing station, the open wards, to the solarium, a flood of memories and feelings brought me back to my residency and attending days. Gordy had a legion of volunteer medical students filming the day. Chicago author and icon Studs Terkel was the keynote speaker.

I listened to the stories told in the solaria by generation after generation of former County physicians. They all had a familiar ring to them because they were the same stories. The same indignities. The same glories. The moments of hope and the episodes of despair. We all still had the "County bug!" It was frightening how little had changed.

The high point of the day was the tour of the new facility. Bright, light and clean, with single and double patient rooms, it was what we had wanted all along—a dignified place to take care of patients. We marveled at the wonder of telephones, toilets and showers in each patient's room and the lack of open wards. A far cry from the tired "Old Lady on Harrison Street." The day concluded with speeches and a photo on bleachers that had been set up in Pasteur Park with the backdrop of County Hospital as the focal point.

I was reminded of the battlefield reunions for the survivors of Pearl Harbor and Normandy. In many ways there were similarities between those vets and us: the camaraderie that comes from shared adversity; the emotional highs and lows that accompany the transition from youth to adulthood, especially those transitions forged in the battleground-like conditions at Cook County Hospital. But unlike soldiers who fight to defend their country, our service was distinct. At County Hospital, our battleground was not a sliver of land, not an Omaha Beach beachhead. At County, the lives of the downtrodden, the rejected, and the dejected were in our hands. As I surveyed the crowd and saw familiar faces, I was buoyed by the medical expertise that surrounded me. County made us better doctors. The war, which felt unwinnable at the time—to keep the hospital open—finally seemed to have been won with the opening of the new facility. A victory which we savored as we basked on bleachers in the afternoon sun while a photo was taken of all of us in front of the battle-scarred old hospital. But beneath the surface of this glorious day a deeper question loomed. Will the new facility alone mean better service and better care for the patients? As we broke up at the end of the day little did we realize that just beyond the horizon were dark clouds that would once again threaten the County Hospital and its patients in an existential way.

CHAPTER 23

2008: *"Déjà Vu All Over Again"*

I STARED AT THE EMPTY MAIN building of the old Cook County Hospital, barely a football field from where I stood on a walkway over Harrison Street at Rush University Hospital. County stood silent and shuttered, more dingy and battered than I remembered. She stretched the whole block of Harrison from Wood to Ogden. The "Old Lady on Harrison Street."

In 2005 I began a new position at Rush University Medical Center, the former Presbyterian Hospital. I came to Rush, across the street from the old County Hospital, in part because of its proximity to and teaching relationship with County Hospital. On this particular day, I lingered a little longer than usual to take in the view in front of me. It was raining. No, it was pouring; not unusual for Chicago in the fall. The warmth of the walkway belied the chill of the pelting rain drumming against the window, inches from my face. From my vantage point, five stories above the street, I peered as far down Harrison Street as I could see, from California to Western to Damen to Ogden, the crossroads of forgotten inner-city neighborhoods that most commuters simply plowed past. Factories with water-tower crowns and the two-flat tenements of Chicago's vast West Side hugged the horizon, not like the majestic high-rises that graced the lakeshore to the east, but plain, unpretentious, stolid structures, homes to plain, unpretentious people. I traced the glistening tracks of cars and trucks pummeling east-bound in a sodden morning rush hour toward a Loop neighborhood far more glamorous than the one I was facing. Then I looked once again at the old Hospital, the veteran of the Chicago health care wars, now a silent sentinel.

Abandoned for six years, it awaited a conversion into administrative offices. On closer inspection, old County was in bad shape, an eyesore. Her crumbling cornices, cracked and dirty, were splinted with metal trusses. These trusses held back loose brick and gargoyles that threatened to hurtle themselves to Harrison Street below in a biblical display. Her façade, with Beaux-Arts carvings, soot-covered bricks and ply-wooded windows, looked forlorn. I had come to County as an idealistic young doctor to work there and change the health care world. Many of us fought against great odds to improve health care delivery for the patients. As I gazed at the crumbling old hospital I was sad to know the dreams and ideals we had to transform the place were not yet close to being realized.

This would have been the perfect place to end this coming-of-age story: the making of a doctor amid the drama and despair of Cook County Hospital; the politics of health care in Chicago; race conflict and health inequity; then a return to the "scene of the crime" years later. But, not so fast. A phone call changed that plan. "Would you be willing to serve on the new Independent Board of Directors for the County Health System if appointed?" the President of the Chicago Medical Society enquired. "You have been nominated."

After leaving County, I spent ten years at Mount Sinai Hospital, an urban teaching hospital smack dab in North Lawndale, one of the poorest urban communities in America. Out from under the shadow of County Hospital, I developed a deeper perspective on health in Chicago and the relationship of race, poverty and mortality. What was causing black people in Chicago to die at higher rates than white people? And at higher rates than in the rest of the U.S.? How could these inequities exist in a modern American city? With all the advances in health care over the past fifty years? I was struck by the plethora of health care institutions in or near the city (including four magnificent academic medical centers), and yet aware of the contradiction that racial health disparities in the city were getting worse. How could that be? I reflected on my seventeen-year sojourn at County Hospital and how that health system contributed to the perpetuation of health care inequities in Chicago because the demand for services was always more than the capacity. The wait lists were too long. The services were not available in the far-flung communities where the patients lived. As a result, late-stage disease was more the norm than the exception, and people died as a result. In ones and twos, but they added up until the racial disparity in mortality in Chicago was one of the highest reported in the nation. This disparity stood out as an indictment of the public and private health care systems that, by design, were failing the city's most vulnerable populations.

Working in Lawndale forced me to reflect on the structure of Chicago's communities and their contribution to poor health. Hyper-segregation and poverty in Chicago contributed to a deterioration of health in many communities. Poor health was not just the result of random acts, bad luck, bad behavior or unfortunate genetics. Deliberate public policy decisions about housing, education, parks and streets were the key drivers of racial differences in mortality. Crime kept people off the streets and limited their ability to exercise. The lack of grocery stores limited dietary choices. The lack of primary care doctors and specialists in these communities made chronic disease care more difficult. The degradation and loss of hospital services in these communities affected hospital-based outcomes. When any health disaster struck Chicago—diabetes, AIDS or breast cancer—these communities suffered a disproportionate amount of the morbidity and mortality. The chronic underfunding of critical health services at Cook County Hospital and other safety-net providers contributed to these poor outcomes as well. The deleterious impact of social structures such as urban poverty and racism on health has been called "structural violence."

The Sinai Urban Health Institute performed door-to-door surveys on health in communities like Lawndale and found epidemic proportions of diabetes, hypertension, smoking, depression, asthma and obesity. The rates among blacks and Latinos were many times higher than among whites in Chicago. The consequence was higher death rates for minorities in Chicago. By 2010, over three thousand black people died every year in Chicago because they did not have the same health care experience as white people. And the inadequacies of the health-care safety net—particularly the County Health System—was partially responsible for this gap. This was not preordained. Much of this was preventable.

The County Health System was plunged into crisis again in 2006. While corruption, poor management and political patronage were blamed, at the heart of this crisis was the growing numbers of uninsured in the Chicago area and the dwindling fiscal support for the public health system. The crisis in 2006 was similar to the one that rocked County Hospital in the late 1970s during my residency. Routine services like screening mammograms had been unavailable for years. Cancer diagnostic services such as colposcopy for cervical cancer or colonoscopy for colon cancer had huge wait lists. Cancer surgeries were delayed. These were diseases amenable to early detection and treatment and the delays contributed to early deaths. Care was rationed in other areas as well. In 2007, almost 100 million dollars in funding and programs were slashed. Longstanding well-regarded community programs, including some I had helped establish years before, were shut down. Hundreds of health care workers were laid off. Many years of hard-fought gains were lost in one year. As in the 1970s, the doctors and nurses organized demonstrations to protest the cuts. The *Chicago Tribune* editorialized against the incompetence of the Cook County Board for allowing patronage hiring and fiscal ineptitude. A Blue Ribbon panel, calling for the formation of an independent board, also pointed out the structural nature of the deficit. The system required more funding. Larger cuts loomed in 2008 if nothing was done. County attending physicians like Mardge Cohen and Gordy Schiff could not bear to witness the further destruction and devastation of the institution they loved. They departed, as did other talented physicians. The public health community in Chicago was in an uproar. It was as if County's heart had been ripped out.

The Cook County Boardroom was packed to the rafters, just like in the old days, crammed with commissioners, union activists, doctors, reporters and other spectators. Budget hearings had been held around the County in the month before. Thousands showed up to testify to the negative health impact of the cuts: the largest turnouts since the 1970s. Many were veterans of the fight for the rebuilding of County Hospital two decades earlier. Some were new to political activism. It was the eleventh hour. The Commissioners were squabbling; the pressure was on. The budget had to be passed that night. Without more funding, the County Health System would lose another 100 million dollars in 2008. Morale was low, despair high. At midnight, a compromise was reached. In exchange for a yes vote by holdout Commissioner, Larry Suffredin, on a sales tax increase that would provide the needed revenues, the County Board President agreed to create an eleven-member Independent Board to run the health system. The first Independent Board in thirty years.

The County Board President was given a list of 84 names of people who had agreed to serve if selected. I was one of them. He did not choose me the first time. But as a few of the first candidates dropped off, I received the nod. After a hearing down at the County Board hearing rooms, where we had held so many protests years before, I was approved. The same battles for health equity that had brought me to County in the seventies were yet to be won. Now I was on the board, there was a new opportunity to make the system work.

I walked down Harrison Street to attend my first Board meeting in the John Stroger Hospital, the new County hospital which stood behind the shuttered Old Lady. Past the locked front entrance of the old hospital, enclosed now by an eight-foot silver chain-link barrier erected to keep the homeless out. How many tragedies and triumphs had those darkened portals witnessed since 1916? On my right in Pasteur Park, there was a grassy space where the Greek restaurant used to be before it burned down. A tattered yellow windsock fluttered inside the fenced-in heliport at the center of the park. I turned the corner on Ogden and Harrison, past the same Fantus Clinic where I spent so much time learning to be a doctor. It looked the worse for wear thirty years later. At the corner, near the sidewalk by the clinic, I saw a familiar face. It was George, the homeless schizophrenic, who first made his home here in the late 1970s. He was wrapped in three or four layers of clothes and was smoking a cigarette. The gray of his matted dreadlocked hair and beard matched mine. I had not seen him in fifteen years.

"Hi George!" I chirped, with a bit too much enthusiasm.

He startled. Shaken from his reveries, he muttered and shook an angry fist in my direction. For George, it was just another day with his demons. I continued down the path to the new hospital entrance and held my breath as I passed the gauntlet of smokers who puffed away by the front door just as they always had. Streams of blue-gray smoke wafted upwards and dissipated. I strode inside to the elevators and met a green-uniformed housekeeper, with a mop in hand. I recognized him. It had been almost fifteen years since I had seen him. He nodded in acknowledgment.

"Hey, didn't you used to work here?" he asked.

"Yeah," I responded. "A long time ago."

The creation of a new independent Board of Directors for the Cook County Health System was a necessary but not sufficient step on the path to improve health for the poor in Chicago. Despite the passage of health reform in 2010, the expectations for its impact on the patients who used County Hospital and its services were low. Unlike Medicare, the government-run elderly health care insurance plan in the U.S. which provides the same coverage to all Americans regardless of race and income, the new reform legislation preserved the caste system of health care in America, one that all but guarantees different health outcomes depending on the patient's insurance status. At least twenty-five million people in the U.S. will remain uninsured and shut out of the private health system. In the Chicago area, up to

500,000 would continue to have no insurance. Those of us who supported single-payer health insurance as the fairest and cheapest way to cover the fifty million uninsured in the U.S. were disappointed. If as Albert Einstein once said, "The definition of insanity is continuing to do the same thing over and over again and expecting a different result," the U.S. health system was an exercise in madness.

What about the future of the Cook County Health System and other public hospital systems across the country? Public hospitals like County will still be the last refuge for the medically deprived in the U.S. Because the tiered system of health care in the U.S. excludes the uninsured from the mainstream, the Cook County Hospitals of the country will always be required to be the last resort for the poor. Public hospitals have always provided some services as well or better than their private counterparts. In Chicago the Emergency, Trauma, Burn, Correctional Health, public health and the services for people with substance abuse and AIDS were a few examples. But for other services, including early disease detection and timely access to specialty care, the public system has fallen short.

With adequate funding and management, there probably is no better equipped provider of health-care delivery for the poor. Community-based clinics providing primary care and specialty care in convenient locations woven into a network of care that allows for the treatment of complex disease in hospitalized settings makes a lot of sense, but has never been adequately resourced in Chicago.

But it is not enough just to save the County Health System, once again, if it is just to preserve an unhappy status quo of poor service and cutbacks. We have to transform the public system to be as good as the best of its private counterparts on all measures of service and outcomes. When this happens, everyone, not just the poor, will seek out care at public health sites for their convenience and quality. That is a tall order for the County Health System. Few public systems across the U.S. have achieved this. Hope lies in a new strategic plan for health that calls for the expansion of primary and specialty care across Cook County, targeting those communities with the worst health results. This plan is just the latest dream for revival of this tottering public health system which has seen many heralded plans for improvement come and go in the last 160 years. At this writing, its future is still unsure as we enter, once again, a dark period of underfunding and cutbacks.

A viable public-health system is still necessary after all these years. But fixing Cook County Hospital is tinkering around the edges until the U.S. adopts a single-payer or similar health insurance program, one that provides equal access to all residents regardless of income, race or ethnicity. Without it we will never succeed at achieving health equity—fairness, equality and dignity for all patients—in Chicago or the U.S. Such a basic human value, so widely accepted across all the major Western industrialized nations of the world except the U.S. Not radical medicine, but common sense. The idea of fairness in health care brought my friends and me to Cook County Hospital in 1978. It was a goal we were not yet close to achieving.

In the park across Harrison Street from the shuttered old County Hospital, there stands a statue of Louis Pasteur, the renowned French physician and humanitarian. On it is a brass plaque, blackened with time from exposure to the harsh Chicago winters and brutal summer heat, on which Pasteur's words are inscribed. They speak to the spirit and possibility that a fair system of health-care delivery holds out to those with the least in our society.

"One doesn't ask of one who suffers: What is your country and what is your religion. One merely says, you suffer, this is enough for me. You belong to me and I will help you."

Words like Pasteur's inspired many young physicians like me to come to Chicago's Cook County Hospital over the last century and a half. Unfortunately, the inhumanity of health injustice still persists. The war we came to Chicago to fight so many years ago rages on. It is a war we have yet to win.

Acknowledgments

I COULD NOT HAVE WRITTEN this book were it not for the collective achievements of the many doctors, nurses and other health-care workers, past and present, who struggled to provide the most basic medical care to the medically indigent of Cook County over the last one hundred and sixty years. While these are my words, the tapestry that comprises the narrative of Cook County Hospital was woven by countless hands.

I must recognize the singular contributions of my wife and life partner, Dr. Paula Grabler, who has been a witness to all the events in this book. We married just after college and she heard the stories that make up this book when they happened and has been subjected to them many times over as this book unfolded over the past seven years. She has been my confidant, pointed with her critiques, and a tireless listener and editor. When we moved to Chicago, she was a social worker whose friends were all training at Cook County Hospital. In her mid thirties, with two small children, she made a bold career change to become a doctor, which included student rotations and an internship at County Hospital. I am indebted to her for her endless love and support.

I wish to thank my parents, and my children, Jonah and Leah. Jonah, the real writer in the family, read this work and delivered unflinching feedback. Through his production company, JAMS, he has overseen the development of a website for the book and has provided countless hours of advice and support. Leah, my medical student daughter, came up with the title for the book, which after months of discarded alternatives, was the obvious choice. My dad, the late Gerald J.E. Ansell, MD, and my mother Phyllis, came to the United States, leaving behind England and socialized medicine, and then raised a son who became a proponent of it. I became a doctor because of them. My parents' steadfast belief in doing the right thing helped me to develop into the doctor I have become.

There are others who deserve mention. Dr. Quentin Young, who wrote the introduction, inspired us to come to Chicago and has been an unrelenting advocate for social justice in health for the past sixty years. My friend and colleague, Steven Whitman, PhD, whose leadership of the Sinai Urban Health Institute and our work together on many projects and countless hours of conversation, has given me deeper insight into the problem of racism and health inequity in Chicago and what needs to be done to fix it.

I want to thank Dr. Larry Goodman, CEO of Rush University Medical Center, a former County doctor himself, for his generous support of me and this endeavor; Drs. Gordy Schiff, David Goldberg and Peter Orris, who answered my desperate calls for photos and reference materials; Mrs. Ruth Rothstein, former CEO of the Cook County Health System; Mrs. Pearlie Bolden, Secretary of the House Staff Association at Cook County Hospital; and Ms. Heather Stecklein of the Rush University Archives for their assistance and access to the County Hospital archives.

I am indebted to author Susan Messer who provided writing and editing guidance to this neophyte author; to Jade Dell for her meticulous editing; to Jordan and Anita Miller of Academy Chicago Publishers for their editorial guidance, graciousness and enthusiasm for this book; to Joan Sommers for her excellent book design; and to Mark Crispin Miller for his untiring efforts to bring the book to the attention of key media.

Finally, I must acknowledge my patients, who allowed a young doctor a window into their lives, their illnesses and their struggles for decency and fairness.

Sources

Books

Bonner, Thomas Neville. *Medicine in Chicago, 1850–1950, A Chapter in the Social and Scientific Development of a City*, 2nd ed., Urbana and Chicago, IL: University of Illinois Press, 1991.

Dowling, Harry F. *City Hospitals: The Undercare of the Underprivileged.* Cambridge, MA: Harvard University Press, 1982.

Lewis, Sydney. *Hospital: An Oral History of Cook County Hospital.* New York: New Press, 1995.

Raffensperger, John G. *The Old Lady On Harrison Street, Cook County Hospital, 1833–1995.* New York: Peter Lang Publishing, 1997.

Archives

Archives, Rush University Medical Center

Archives, House Staff Association, John H. Stroger, Jr. Hospital of Cook County

Photo Archives, John H. Stroger, Jr. Hospital of Cook County

Archives, *Chicago Tribune*

Index